THE 30-MINUTE RENAL DIET COOKBOOK

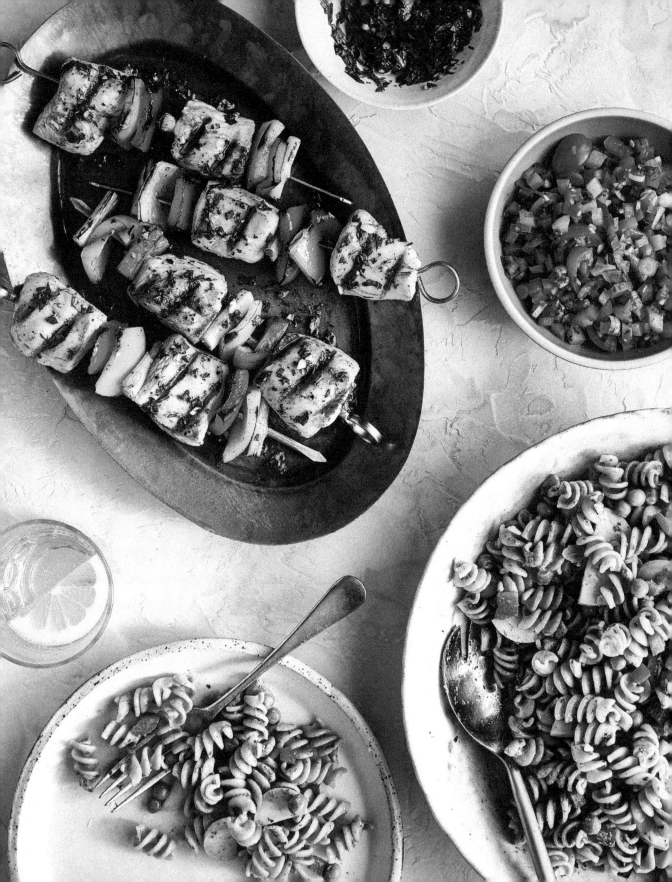

the 30-Minute
RENAL
DIET
COOKBOOK

Easy, Flavorful Recipes for
Every Stage of Kidney Disease

AISLING WHELAN, MS, RDN, CDN

ROCKRIDGE
PRESS

For general information on our other products and services or to obtain technical support, please contact our Customer Care Department within the United States at (866) 744-2665, or outside the United States at (510) 253-0500.

Rockridge Press publishes its books in a variety of electronic and print formats. Some content that appears in print may not be available in electronic books, and vice versa.

Interior and Cover Designer: Heather Krakora
Art Producer: Maura Boland
Editor: Britt Bogan
Production Editor: Jenna Dutton

Photography © 2019 Helene Dujardin, Food styling by Tammi Haberman

Author photo courtesy of ©Andee Maher.

Cover recipe: Turkey Pho (page 119)

ISBN: Print   978-1-64152-696-8
        eBook 978-1-64152-697-5

This book is dedicated to my mother, Margaret, and my husband, Brian. Your support, guidance, and encouragement meant the world to me on this journey.

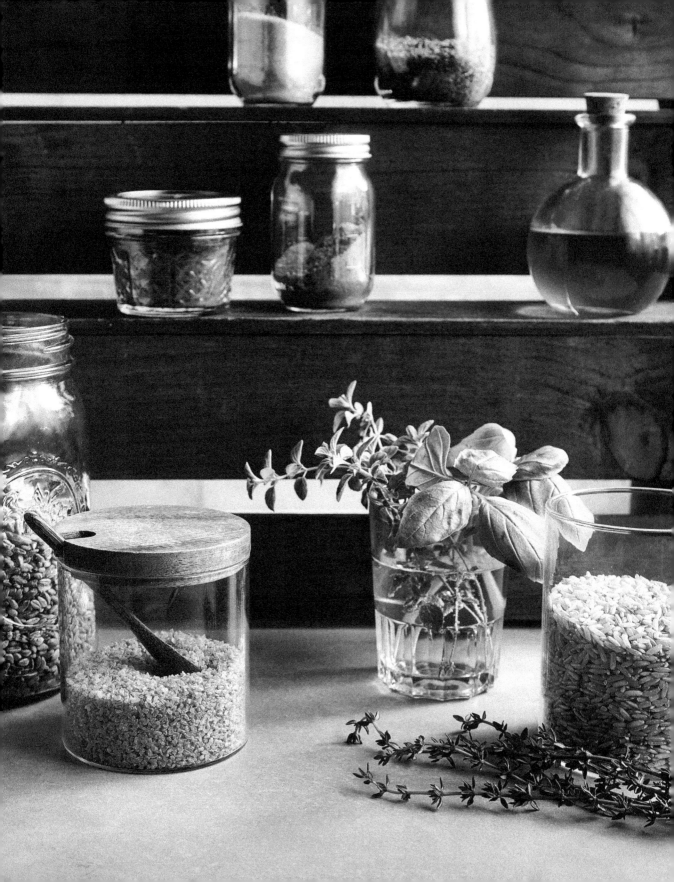

Contents

Introduction

CHRONIC Kidney Disease (CKD) affects 26 million Americans and an estimated 10 percent of the population worldwide. If you're reading this book, chances are that you or someone you love is among those affected, and you're looking for help. You've come to the right place! Nutrition is a powerful weapon in the fight against CKD, and this book has everything you need to harness that power. According to the National Institute of Health, diet therapy can slow the progression of CKD. It almost seems too good to be true. You might worry that achieving results means giving up all of your favorite foods and commiting to a bland, tasteless diet forever. As a renal dietitian who works with CKD patients every day, I can tell you that it doesn't have to be this way. You can improve your health and quality of life by eating foods that are both nourishing *and delicious!*

Typically, when I see a new patient, I find that their knowledge of the renal diet has come from a handout at the doctor's office or from the Internet. While good-quality online resources can be incredibly useful, many sites portray the renal diet as a minefield of contradictions and confusion. Recommendations are sometimes outdated and not always suitable for a patient's particular disease stage and individual needs. Most doctors, while well-meaning, don't have enough time to educate their patients on the renal diet, and so they rely on educational handouts that usually consist of long lists of foods *not* to eat. Instead of feeling empowered, patients are left feeling anxious that there's nothing they *can* eat.

For my patients with diabetes, this confusion and anxiety around what to eat is all too common. They often express frustration at how diabetic nutritional recommendations seem to contradict CKD nutritional recommendations. One patient shared, "I thought I was doing the right thing by switching to whole grains, but then I heard that whole grains are bad for my kidneys." Another patient with hypertension expressed, "I began eating lots of fruits and vegetables to help my blood pressure, but now I'm worried about eating too much potassium." Besides confusion about what to eat, many of my patients report feeling burdened by the amount of time and expense involved in preparing healthy recipes. With all of these frustrations, is it any wonder that the renal diet is perceived as daunting and stressful?

Nutrition counseling can clear up the confusion surrounding these topics in a couple of sessions. Instead of feeling frustrated and anxious, patients begin to feel confident and motivated in their ability to make the changes necessary for their health. Recently, one of my patients shared that he had his first "successful" doctor visit in a long time. He was delighted that understanding and following the renal diet led to significantly improved lab values. This book's purpose is to share with you the wisdom I've gathered from my experience working with patients across the full spectrum of CKD. This book contains delicious, health-promoting, budget-friendly recipes tailored to meet the needs of patients with every stage of CKD. In addition to recipes, this book will give you the information you'll need to make calculated healthy decisions when planning your daily meals. In most cases, the number of ingredients won't be overwhelming (some will have as few as five), and the meals can be rustled up in 30 minutes or less. So, without further ado, let's get cooking!

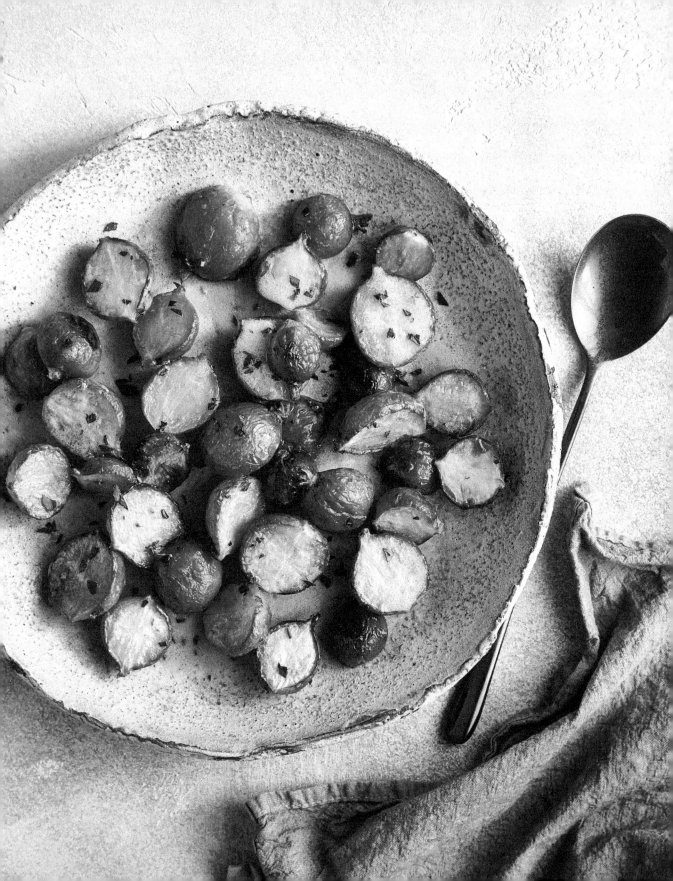

The Renal Diet Made Simple

HOW often do we hear that we need to advocate for our own health? I totally agree we should. But advocating for yourself shouldn't just mean asking your doctor the right questions. To me, it means using trustworthy sources to educate yourself about your condition so you can discover the most effective tools to fight or manage it.

This chapter outlines what chronic kidney disease (CKD) is and explains how the renal diet supports kidney function. We'll discuss both the types of foods you may need to limit and the ones to focus on including in your diet. To fully inform you about the diet's critical impact on your CKD progression, I may get a little "sciencey" on occasion. Understanding how the renal diet affects your body will help you learn how to make the diet work best for you.

⇦*Roasted Radishes, page 45*

MANAGING KIDNEY DISEASE THROUGH DIET

What Is Chronic Kidney Disease?

A CKD diagnosis means that someone's kidneys are experiencing a gradual loss of function. This loss of function usually occurs over months or years, and it often goes undetected in the early stages. For this reason, kidney disease is called a "silent disease." Your doctor evaluates you for CKD by performing several tests. One of these tests, a urine analysis, measures the amount of protein in your urine. Finding protein in urine is abnormal, and it can be indicative of kidney damage. Another kidney function test assesses your *glomerular filtration rate* (GFR). GFR measures how much blood filters through your kidneys each minute. In general, the lower the GFR, the more advanced the kidney disease. If GFR drops to below 15, a person is considered to be in renal failure, also known as end-stage renal disease. When end-stage renal disease is diagnosed, kidney function has declined to the point where dialysis is required, or a kidney transplant is necessary for survival.

What Causes CKD?

While CKD can have many possible causes, diabetes and hypertension most commonly lead to its development. Diabetes is a condition characterized by excessive sugar in the blood, and hypertension is a condition characterized by excessive pressure in the blood. The kidneys' filtering units, known as *nephrons*, are very sensitive to the effects of excessive sugar and pressure. Over time, if these conditions are not controlled, they can contribute to both the development and progression of CKD.

How the Renal Diet Supports Kidney Function

Some of the key drivers of CKD include chronic inflammation and acid build-up (*acidosis*), which hasten the progression of CKD over time. If you have CKD and are not on dialysis, your top priority is likely slowing down CKD progression. Diet can play a powerful role in this because many foods have naturally anti-inflammatory and acid-neutralizing properties.

When it comes to supporting kidney function, wholesome plant foods are essential to include. Practically speaking, this category includes minimally processed foods of plant origin, such as fruits, vegetables, legumes, and olive oil. If inflammation is a fire, wholesome plant foods—readily available at your local grocery store—are the fire extinguishers. In addition to their anti-inflammatory compounds, many wholesome plant foods are also good sources of prebiotics, which we can think of as dinner for the trillions of bacteria residing in our gut. An imbalance of friendly and unfriendly bacteria in the gut, known as *dysbiosis*, is thought to influence CKD progression by increasing inflammation. In addition to reducing inflammation, wholesome plant foods are also the antidote for the acidosis that occurs as CKD progresses. By incorporating more wholesome plant foods in your diet, you can neutralize the acid build-up and enhance the health of your gut, which, in turn, will improve the health of your kidneys.

RENAL DIET GUIDELINES

An individualized renal diet works in various ways to support your remaining kidney function. This section reviews the renal diet guidelines, focusing on the nutrients that you may need to limit, as well as pointers to help you make smart choices for managing your CKD.

Manage Your Intake of Key Nutrients

There are several important nutrients to consider when planning an individualized renal diet. The stage of your CKD, your individual lab values, and your other coexisting conditions will help determine how these nutrients should fit into your renal diet. Before making any dietary changes, I encourage you to consult with your healthcare provider (HCP) for more specific recommendations based on your unique health situation.

POTASSIUM

Managing potassium can sometimes be confusing because intake recommendations can change as CKD progresses. When we eat potassium, an electrolyte essential for many bodily functions, our body uses what's needed and excretes what's not. As kidney function declines, the kidneys become less efficient at removing potassium through the urine. Potassium can build up in the blood when it isn't excreted properly, leading to a potentially dangerous condition called *hyperkalemia*. This is more likely to occur in the later stages of CKD.

In CKD stages 1 to 3, the kidneys usually retain their ability to excrete extra potassium, so restricting potassium is typically unnecessary. Many wholesome plant foods are rich in potassium. According to a study published in the *British Journal of Medicine*, high dietary potassium intake is linked with lowering the risk of conditions like stroke and hypertension. Since eating potassium-rich foods is beneficial, and since many people with CKD can still excrete potassium effectively, renal nutrition guidelines recommend that dietary potassium be adjusted to maintain a potassium blood level within the normal range. This means that you should restrict potassium only if your health care provider determines that it is necessary to maintain a normal blood level of potassium. See the Food Lists for the Renal Diet on page 155 for foods' potassium content.

PROTEIN

For those with CKD who are not on dialysis, the amount of protein consumed can affect how quickly CKD progresses. Eating too much protein should be avoided, as it makes the kidneys work harder to process it. I tell my CKD patients to think of lowering their diet's protein intake as a way of giving their kidneys a rest. Decreasing dietary protein intake has been shown to improve certain physical measures of CKD, such as protein in the urine. Also, according to a systematic review published by the Academy of Nutrition and Dietetics, current research suggests that people with CKD who lower their protein consumption may be able to slow CKD progression and improve their overall longevity and quality of life.

Like potassium, protein is a nutrient that requires a lot of individualization, so determining how much is too much will depend on your stage of CKD, your body size, your height, and your unique health situation. The table on page 12 will help you estimate your daily protein needs, and as always, you should consult with your health care provider for additional guidance.

If you need to lower your protein consumption, a plant-based diet is one of the easiest ways to achieve this. Since most plant-derived foods naturally contain less protein than animal-derived foods, a plant-based diet reduces the amount of protein in your diet without making you feel deprived. A plant-based diet is not the same thing as a vegetarian or vegan diet. While some people with CKD may choose to become vegetarians or vegans, this approach may not be desirable or achievable for everyone. This cookbook advocates a plant-based diet that still includes animal-derived foods, but in smaller portions and less frequently, such as at one meal per day.

If you are on dialysis and need to increase the amount of protein you eat, chances are, this won't be a significant adjustment to your current diet. The standard American diet already contains more protein than the amount required for health. However, getting enough protein may become tricky if you are experiencing a decreased appetite or unpleasant symptoms, such as nausea or fatigue. These issues can make eating and preparing meals more challenging. Malnutrition is a common concern for people on dialysis, and this can negatively impact their prognosis and quality of life. A renal dietitian can help you manage these issues and may prescribe dietary changes or dietary supplements to prevent malnutrition. See page 158 for a list of the protein content of various foods.

PHOSPHORUS

For most people with CKD, dietary phosphorus is a new concept. Managing phosphorus intake is essential during every stage of CKD to prevent serious renal complications, such as renal bone disease (weak and brittle bones) and cardiovascular disease. While this may sound alarming, successfully managing phosphorus intake is entirely possible. What's important to take away from this section is that the source of phosphorus matters.

There are three different sources of phosphorus in the diet: (1) plant-protein foods, such as whole grains, legumes, and nuts; (2) animal-protein foods, such as meat, cheese, and fish; and (3) phosphorus additives, which is the phosphorus added to processed foods and beverages, such as canned and bottled drinks, frozen meals, and many other packaged foods. See page 9 for guidance on how to look for phosphorus additives and preservatives in foods and beverages.

The source of phosphorus matters because, depending on the source, your body's ability to absorb it can vary tremendously. This variation in how much of a nutrient is absorbed from a particular food is called *bioavailability*. When a person with CKD eats a diet with highly bioavailable forms of phosphorus, their body absorbs most of the phosphorus they are eating. The more bioavailable phosphorus someone eats, the more at risk they are of experiencing some of the negative complications associated with phosphorus. But before we go any further, let's get something straight. Which source of phosphorus is the most bioavailable, and which source is the least? According to a study published in the *Journal of Renal Nutrition*, the absorption of phosphorus varies widely depending on the type of food. If I had a red carpet, I would be rolling it out for wholesome plant foods about now. That's because wholesome plant foods are the stars when it comes to phosphorus. Estimates suggest that the absorption rate can sometimes be as low as 10 percent for the phosphorus found in plant foods and as high as 100 percent for the phosphorus added to processed foods. The absorption of phosphorus in animal foods like meat and dairy is estimated to be somewhere in the middle. Clearly, no red carpet for the additives!

Since phosphorus is not listed on most food labels or in most recipes, I tell my patients to look at the sources of phosphorus in their diet. The best way to control your phosphorus intake is to eat an abundance of plant foods, a moderate amount of animal foods, and as little phosphorus additives as possible. Phosphorus control tends to be most challenging for people on dialysis, as, at this stage, the kidney's ability to excrete phosphorus is most impaired. Additionally, people on dialysis sometimes need to increase their intake of higher phosphorus animal foods, such as meat and dairy, to meet their daily protein requirements. Many people on dialysis benefit from a medication, called a phosphorus binder, to help keep their phosphorus level under control. The list starting on page 161 shows the phosphorus content of various foods.

Limit Your Sodium Intake

Sodium is a mineral and an electrolyte that we obtain through our diet. When consumed in excessive amounts, it can contribute to high blood pressure, a significant risk factor for cardiovascular disease and stroke. High blood pressure is a common concern for people with CKD, and it tends to escalate as CKD progresses. For this reason, the higher your stage of CKD, the more "salt sensitive" you are likely to be. Limiting your sodium intake can help control your blood pressure and help manage symptoms such as fluid retention (a side effect of high sodium intake). According to an article published in the journal *BMC Nephrology*, a low-protein diet combined with sodium restriction can reduce the amount of protein in the urine, a marker of kidney damage.

For people with CKD (at any stage), the recommended sodium intake is 2300 milligrams per day, which is equivalent to about 1 teaspoon of salt. If this seems like a lot to you, you might be surprised to learn that most Americans exceed this amount daily. "Hidden salt" in processed foods and restaurant meals represents the majority of dietary sodium. According to the American Heart Association, processed foods and restaurant foods contribute 71 percent of Americans' sodium intake. Salt added in cooking accounts for only 6 percent, while salt added at the table accounts for a mere 5 percent. Therefore, cutting back on processed foods and how often you eat out is the best way to keep your sodium intake within the recommended limits.

Since it isn't practical or necessary to avoid all processed foods, make a habit of checking sodium on the nutrition label. Many canned, frozen, jarred, and packaged foods are available as low-sodium or with no added salt. Cooking most of your meals at home helps you avoid high sodium restaurant foods. Dining out is still possible on a low-sodium diet. The "Food Lists for the Renal Diet" section on page 155 lists the sodium content of common foods.

Choose High-Fiber Carbohydrates

When thinking about carbohydrates, it's helpful to group them into two different types: refined carbohydrates and unrefined carbohydrates. Refined carbohydrates include food and beverages such as sugar-sweetened drinks, pastries, white bread, and candy. Unrefined carbohydrates include vegetables, fruit, legumes, and whole grains. When refined carbohydrates predominate your diet, the risk of inflammation is higher, and this can trigger chronic health conditions such as obesity, diabetes, and cardiovascular disease. Unrefined carbohydrate foods, on the other hand, contribute fiber to your diet, an important dietary component for health. People who consume high-fiber diets tend to have a more favorable balance of friendly and unfriendly bacteria in the gut, which is beneficial for people with CKD. While whole grains were traditionally discouraged on a renal diet, due to their higher potassium and phosphorus content, modern renal recommendations recognize the benefits of including them. Whole grains contain the least bioavailable form of phosphorus, and while there are certain exceptions, most whole grains provide only a marginal amount of extra potassium compared to refined grains. See "Food Lists for the Renal Diet" for examples of high-fiber carbohydrates.

CARBOHYDRATES AND DIABETES

If you have diabetes, limiting your intake of refined carbohydrates is crucial, as these foods tend to have the most significant impact on blood sugar. Your healthcare provider may advise that you eat a specific amount of carbohydrates at each meal and snack. Refer to page 10 for guidance on how to determine the number of carbohydrates in a particular food. Many of the recipes in this book are considered diabetic-friendly or include a diabetes tip to help adjust the recipe to your needs.

Use Heart-Healthy Fats

When it comes to fats, let's make one thing clear: The renal diet is not a low-fat diet! Don't think of fat as the enemy; the heart-healthy kind of fat is your friend. Heart-healthy fats add flavor and richness to your meals, while also greatly benefiting your health. Olive oil is an excellent example. According to a study published in the journal *BMC Medicine*, olive oil consumption is associated with a lower risk of developing cardiovascular disease. The benefits of olive oil are thought to be due to its high content of anti-inflammatory polyphenols and oleic acid. Avocado oil has similar properties to olive oil, and it is a popular cooking choice due to its high smoke point and mild flavor. Other examples of heart-healthy fats include the omega-3 fatty acids found in certain fish like salmon and mackerel, along with the omega-6 fatty acids found in nut butters such as almond or peanut butter.

The primary dietary fats you'll want to avoid are the trans fats. Trans fats are found in processed foods that contain partially hydrogenated oil. (Look for this in the ingredients section.) The American Heart Association recommends avoiding trans fats, as research has linked their consumption to a higher risk of developing heart disease and stroke. When it comes to saturated fats, found in foods such as butter, coconut oil, and cheese, the research is not as clear. While eating saturated fat has been shown to increase LDL (bad cholesterol), the link between saturated fat and the risk of heart disease remains unproven and hotly debated. If you have CKD and your cholesterol is under control, there is no reason to strictly eliminate saturated fats from your diet. It is much more important to focus on the more relevant nutrients to your condition, as mentioned in the sections above. However, if you do struggle with an elevated LDL, you may need to be more careful about your saturated fat consumption. As always, consult your HCP for further guidance on this topic.

Track Your Fluid Intake

Fluid management is a vital element of the renal diet and is highly individual. Many people with CKD need to drink enough fluids to keep their kidneys hydrated. People on dialysis, however, usually need to restrict their fluid intake to prevent overhydration. Ask your HCP about how much fluid to consume each day, and consider measuring your consumption to ensure you meet your needs.

HOW TO READ NUTRITION LABELS

Nutrition labels are a useful tool for choosing foods suitable for your health and personal needs. Below is a guide to help you read them.

Ingredients: Before looking at the nutrition facts panel, quickly scan the ingredients to see if anything unexpected catches your eye. For example, in a can of lentil soup, are there lentils, vegetables, and seasonings? Take note of strange-sounding additives. This may be red-flag territory. While some additives, such as citric acid, are okay and often necessary for shelf-stable foods, a long list of additives may signal that the food is highly processed. People with CKD need to be cautious of the phosphorus additives used to increase products' shelf life and palatability. Phosphorus additives are commonly added to sodas, enhanced meat products, baked goods, and many other boxed, canned, and packaged foods. Phosphorus additives represent the most bioavailable form of phosphorus in the diet. Below are examples of phosphorus additives used by the food industry:

> **Phosphoric acid**
> **Polyphosphate**
> **Sodium tripolyphosphate**
> **Tricalcium phosphate**
> **Trisodium phosphate**

Serving Size: All of the nutrition information on the label reflects the serving size. If you are eating a smaller or bigger portion than the serving size, you will need to adjust the nutrients accordingly. For example, if the serving size is ½ cup and you eat 1 cup, you will be getting twice the amount of nutrients listed on the label.

Nutrition Facts Panel: The nutrition facts panel contains a lot of information, and some of this information will be more relevant to you based on your personal needs. If you have CKD, be sure to check the following nutrients:

Sodium: 2300 milligrams is the daily recommended amount of sodium for CKD. Think of this as your sodium budget. Every time you eat something that has sodium in it, you are spending some of your budget. So, be vigilant about checking products' sodium content.

Protein: Protein needs vary by individual. Be informed about your individual needs (see page 11) so that a glance at the nutrition labels will show you how the product fits into your daily protein needs.

Fiber: Fiber is the indigestible portion of plant foods found in vegetables, fruits, legumes, and whole grains. It has multiple benefits, and many people don't get enough of it. It is recommended that men take in 38 grams of fiber and women take in 25 grams of fiber each day.

Carbohydrates: If you have diabetes and are counting carbs, you can check the total carbohydrate section of the label. Since fiber is an indigestible carbohydrate that will not affect your blood sugar, you can subtract the fiber from the total carbohydrates to get the net carbs.

Sugar: One thing many of my patients find helpful is that 4 grams of sugar equals 1 teaspoon of sugar. So, if a product has 16 grams of sugar, that amounts to approximately 4 teaspoons of sugar.

Potassium: The potassium content will be listed on all nutrition labels by 2021. Until then, the best way of determining if a food is high in potassium is to look at the ingredients. See page 155 for examples and keep in mind that ingredients on a food label are listed in order of predominance.

Stage-by-Stage Nutritional Needs

CKD STAGE	PROTEIN	SODIUM	POTASSIUM	PHOSPHORUS
1–2	0.8 grams protein per kilogram of ideal body weight	2300 milligrams per day for all stages	Adjust intake to maintain a blood potassium level within the normal range.	Adjust intake to maintain a blood phosphorus level within the normal range.
3–5 (Non-dialysis)	0.55–0.6 grams protein per kilogram of ideal body weight			
Stage 5 Dialysis (All modalities)	1–1.2 grams protein per kilogram of ideal body weight			

FOR DIABETES

If you have diabetes and you have CKD stage 1–5 (not on dialysis) your protein needs are 0.8–0.9 grams per kilogram of ideal body weight.

If you are on dialysis and have diabetes, your protein needs are the same as non-diabetics (1–1.2 grams protein per kilogram of ideal body weight).

ADDITIONAL NOTES

Protein: To calculate your estimated protein needs, find your ideal body weight in the table on page 12 and multiply it by the grams of protein prescribed for your stage.

Example: If you are a male and 5 feet, 8 inches tall with CKD stage 2, your estimated ideal body weight is 70 kilograms. You would calculate your estimated daily protein needs by multiplying 0.8 grams protein by 70 kilograms.

0.8g protein × 70 kilograms = 56 grams protein per day.

Sodium: Consuming less than 1500 milligrams is not recommended as it may increase the risk of complications.

Ideal Body Weight

MALE		FEMALE	
HEIGHT	IBW (KG)	HEIGHT	IBW (KG)
5 ft	48	4 ft 10	41
5 ft 1	51	4 ft 11	43
5 ft 2	54	5 ft	45
5 ft 3	56	5 ft 1	48
5 ft 4	59	5 ft 2	50
5 ft 5	62	5 ft 3	52
5 ft 6	65	5 ft 4	55
5 ft 7	67	5 ft 5	57
5 ft 8	70	5 ft 6	59
5 ft 9	73	5 ft 7	61
5 ft 10	75	5 ft 8	64
5 ft 11	78	5 ft 9	66
6 ft	81	5 ft 10	68
6 ft 1	84	5 ft 11	70
6 ft 2	86	6 ft	73
6 ft 3	89		
6 ft 4	92		

The weights listed in this table provide a quick estimate of your lean body mass. Your ideal body weight may be higher or lower than the weight listed in this table. Many factors go into determining an individual's ideal body weight, and so you should consult your HCP for more specific guidance.

QUICK AND EASY MEALS

Now that you have an understanding of the renal dietary guidelines, you probably have a fair idea of the kinds of foods to include in your diet and the types of foods to limit. To apply this knowledge of the renal diet guidelines in your life, you'll now need to find meals and snacks that you enjoy and are easy to prepare. Enter the renal recipes!

How Our Recipes Help

The recipes in this cookbook are designed to be nourishing and delicious, and to accommodate each stage of CKD. The recipes include different informative tips such as how to modify the ingredients to lower or raise the protein or to make the dish more suitable for someone with diabetes. Convenience is the name of the game here—you won't spend hours in the kitchen! All of the recipes can be completed in 30 minutes or less and the ingredients used are simple and affordable. Some recipes require five ingredients or fewer, and many can be made in one pot, making cleanup a breeze. I hope the recipes in this book help reduce the stress of cooking for yourself, your family, or for someone you take care of—all while you reap the many nutritional benefits.

Practical Tips and Tricks

Embrace leftovers by cooking in bulk. Leftovers allow you the freedom to take a night off from cooking. Store leftovers in the refrigerator for up to 3 to 4 days or freeze them. Use frozen leftovers within 3 to 4 months.

Prep your ingredients. One way to make cooking more manageable is to measure out, wash, and prepare all the ingredients before you start cooking. Taking care of all the prep beforehand allows you to focus solely on the cooking.

Use pre-cut fresh and/or frozen vegetables. Frozen vegetables can save time, especially in recipes containing many vegetables. Choose vegetables without added sauce or seasoning to reduce the sodium content.

Use canned beans and lentils. Beans and lentils can take a long time to prepare, and this can be inconvenient. Canned beans and lentils are a perfect antidote. Look for cans that are labeled BPA-free and have no salt added or are low-sodium.

Use frozen grains. You may find it helpful to batch cook grains and freeze them for later use. You can also purchase pre-cooked, frozen products from the grocery store. Always check frozen items for added salt or phosphorus additives.

Clean as you go. Okay, I know that most people don't enjoy cleaning up, but cleaning as you go makes the task less daunting at the end.

Ensure you have the right tools. The right cooking tools are crucial for cutting prep time, avoiding accidents, and ensuring food safety. Some essentials are a sharp knife for cutting vegetables, cutting boards, measuring cups, and measuring spoons.

Stay on top of your supplies. Keep a dry erase board or chalkboard in your kitchen to keep track of staple ingredients that you are about to run out of. You can then avoid realizing in the middle of a recipe that you are missing one of the key ingredients, such as garlic or olive oil.

Organize your pantry, refrigerator, and freezer so that things are easy to find. A spice rack is great for organizing spices. Glass food storage containers are easy to clean and are ideal for storing ingredients, as well as leftovers in the refrigerator or freezer for later use. Always label and date the containers to help you keep track of what you have on hand and how long it has been there.

Set the mood. Cooking can be a relaxing and enjoyable experience when you create the right environment. Before you start, make sure the kitchen is ready for use. Is the equipment clean and in working condition? Set out all of the ingredients needed. Maybe throw on a chef's hat for fun, and don't forget to crank up your favorite music.

THE KIDNEY-FRIENDLY KITCHEN

Basic Kitchen Equipment

- Baking dish
- Can opener
- Chef's knife
- Cooking thermometer
- Cutting boards
- Measuring cups and spoons
- Paring knife
- Set of pots
- Sheet pan
- Skillet
- Vegetable peeler

Pantry Essentials

FRESH

- Almond milk, unsweetened
- Animal protein such as eggs, fish, turkey, and chicken
- Bread, whole-wheat (look for a brand without phosphate additives)
- Fruit
- Vegetables
- Yogurt, plain

FROZEN

- Frozen berries
- Frozen vegetables

CANNED

- Canned beans
- Canned fish

HERBS, SPICES & BAKING

- Baking soda
- Basil
- Cinnamon
- Cornmeal
- Cornstarch
- Cream of tartar
- Curry powder
- Flour, all-purpose and whole-wheat
- Garlic powder
- Oregano
- Pepper
- Salt
- Thyme
- Vanilla extract

CONTINUED

GRAINS

- Barley
- Brown rice
- Bulgur
- Farro
- Oats
- Puffed rice cereal
- Whole-wheat pasta

MISCELLANEOUS

- Broth, vegetable or chicken, low-sodium
- Mustard, Dijon
- Nuts (pecans, walnuts, macadamia nuts, peanuts)
- Oil, avocado
- Oil, olive
- Peanut butter
- Seeds (flax, chia)
- Soy sauce, low-sodium
- Sweetener (brown sugar, honey, maple syrup, or powdered erythritol, a sugar alternative for diabetes)
- Vinegar, apple cider
- Vinegar, balsamic

Healthy Store-Bought Shortcuts

- Brown rice, frozen
- Fruit canned in 100-percent fruit juice
- Garlic, fresh-peeled
- Lettuce, pre-washed (romaine, baby kale, baby spinach, spring mix, etc.)
- Vegetables, frozen

ABOUT THE RECIPES

The recipes in this book are designed to make following the renal diet easy and enjoyable. All of the recipes in this book contain a low to moderate amount of sodium, potassium, and phosphorus, making them suitable for all stages of CKD. In addition to containing nutritional information, each recipe contains at least one recipe label and one recipe tip. Below is an explanation of the recipe labels and tips.

Recipe Labels

Low Protein: Recipes with this label have less than 15 grams of protein per serving in larger dishes like entrées, and less than 5 grams of protein per serving in smaller dishes like snacks and desserts. If your estimated protein needs fall between 30 and 40 grams per day, you should choose mostly low-protein recipes.

Medium Protein: Recipes with this label have protein that ranges from 15 to 24 grams per serving in larger dishes like entrées, and protein that ranges from 5 to 9 grams per serving in smaller dishes like snacks and desserts. If your estimated protein needs fall between 40 and 60 grams per day, you should choose a combination of low- and medium-protein recipes.

High Protein: Recipes with this label have 25 or more grams of protein per serving in larger dishes like entrées, and 10 or more grams of protein per serving in smaller dishes like snacks and desserts. If your protein needs are 60 grams or more per day, choose a combination of medium- and high-protein recipes.

High Fiber: Recipes with this label have more than 5 grams of fiber per serving in larger dishes like entrées, and more than 2 grams of fiber per serving in smaller dishes like snacks and desserts.

Diabetes-Friendly: This label indicates that the recipe is suitable for people with diabetes.

5 Ingredient: This label indicates that the recipe uses only 5 ingredients or fewer (not counting salt, pepper, or oil).

One Pot: This label indicates that the recipe will only require that you use a single cooking vessel, making cleanup a breeze!

Recipe Tips

Diabetes Tip: Suggests a modification to make the recipe appropriate for people with diabetes.

Increase Protein Tip: Suggests a modification to increase the recipe's protein content, which may make it more appropriate for people on dialysis or for someone who has higher protein needs due to their body size.

Reduce Protein Tip: Suggests a modification to reduce the protein content of the recipe, which may make it more appropriate for someone with CKD stages 3 to 5 (non-dialysis).

Make It Easier Tip: Suggests a modification to make a recipe more convenient/quick to prepare.

Ingredient Tip: Provides information or advice about using a particular ingredient in a recipe.

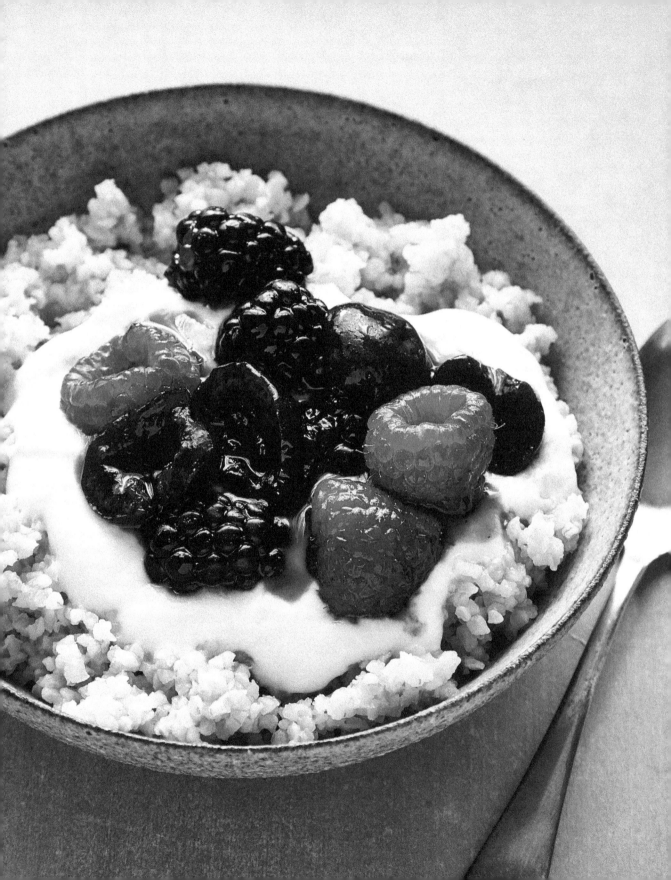

Breakfast

⇦Cherry Berry Bulgur Bowl, page 21

Mixed Berry Smoothie

5-INGREDIENT, HIGH FIBER, LOW PROTEIN

Serves 4 • Prep time: 10 minutes

There are many colorful frozen mixed berry combinations available in the grocery store—strawberries, blackberries, blueberries, raspberries, and more exotic choices such as açaí, boysenberries, and cranberries. Berries are high in anti-oxidants and may reduce inflammation in the body. They're also low in potassium and lower in sugar compared to other fruits.

2 cups mixed
   frozen berries

1½ cups vanilla-flavored
   unsweetened
   almond milk

4 ounces cream
   cheese, softened

½ cup vanilla
   whole-milk yogurt

¼ cup flaxseed

1. Put the berries, almond milk, cream cheese, yogurt, and flaxseed in a blender or food processor. Blend or process until the mixture is smooth.

2. Serve immediately or cover and store in the refrigerator for up to 1 day. The smoothie may separate and be thicker after storage. Just stir it and add a bit more almond milk to get the desired texture.

Increase Protein Tip: To make this a medium-protein recipe, add 1 scoop (2 tablespoons) of unflavored or vanilla protein powder. Adding a protein powder with 30 grams protein per scoop will increase the protein content to 13 grams per serving.

Diabetes Tip: When fruit is blended or juiced, the sugar content is more concentrated. This can lead to blood sugar spikes. To make this a diabetes-friendly recipe, use plain whole-milk yogurt instead of vanilla. The sugar content will decrease to 10 grams per serving. If you desire extra sweetness, add droplets of liquid stevia to taste.

Nutrition Info per Serving: Calories: 249; Total fat: 17g; Saturated fat: 7g; Sodium: 171mg; Phosphorus: 146mg; Potassium: 351mg; Carbohydrates: 21g; Fiber: 6g; Protein: 6g; Sugar: 13g

Cherry Berry Bulgur Bowl

HIGH FIBER, LOW PROTEIN

Serves 4 • Prep time: 15 minutes • Cook time: 15 minutes

Delicious porridge can be made with any grain, including nutty-tasting bulgur. Bulgur is cracked wheat that has been parboiled so it cooks more quickly. This high-fiber grain is an excellent choice for people with CKD. When combined with sweet cherries, colorful berries, and yogurt, it makes a delicious breakfast.

1 cup medium-grind bulgur

2 cups water

Pinch salt

1 cup halved and pitted cherries or 1 cup canned cherries, drained

½ cup raspberries

½ cup blackberries

1 tablespoon cherry jam

2 cups plain whole-milk yogurt

1. In a medium saucepan over medium heat, combine the bulgur, water, and salt. Bring to a boil.

2. Reduce the heat to low and simmer, partially covered, for 12 to 15 minutes or until the bulgur is almost tender. Remove the pan from the heat, cover, and let stand for 5 minutes to finish cooking.

3. While the bulgur is cooking, combine the raspberries and blackberries in a medium bowl. Stir the cherry jam into the fruit.

4. When the bulgur is tender, divide among four bowls. Top each bowl with ½ cup of yogurt and an equal amount of the berry mixture and serve.

Increase Protein Tip: To make this a medium-protein recipe, use nonfat plain Greek yogurt. The amount of protein per serving will increase to 18 grams.

Diabetes Tip: To make this a diabetes-friendly recipe, omit the cherry jam and reduce the cherries in the recipe to ½ cup. The carbohydrates will be reduced to 38 grams per serving (31 net carbs) and the sugar to 9 grams per serving.

Nutrition Info per Serving: Calories: 241; Total fat: 5g; Saturated fat: 3g; Sodium: 85mg; Phosphorus: 237mg; Potassium: 438mg; Carbohydrates: 44g; Fiber: 7g; Protein: 9g; Sugar: 13g

Baked Curried Apple Oatmeal Cups

HIGH FIBER, LOW PROTEIN

Serves 6 • Prep time: 10 minutes • Cook time: 20 minutes

Baked oatmeal has a completely different texture from stovetop-cooked oatmeal. This easy recipe is like a muffin or a soft oatmeal cookie, but denser and more delicious. You can add any fruit to this recipe; blueberries or raspberries would be delicious. If you aren't a fan of curry, use 1 teaspoon cinnamon instead.

Baking spray
3½ cups
   old-fashioned oats
3 tablespoons
   brown sugar

2 teaspoons of your
   preferred curry powder
⅛ teaspoon salt
1 cup unsweetened
   almond milk

1 cup unsweetened
   applesauce
1 teaspoon vanilla
½ cup chopped walnuts

1. Preheat the oven to 375°F. Spray a 12-cup muffin tin with baking spray and set aside.

2. In a medium bowl, combine the oats, brown sugar, curry powder, and salt, and mix.

3. In a small bowl, stir together the milk, applesauce, and vanilla.

4. Stir the liquid ingredients into the dry ingredients and mix until just combined. Stir in the walnuts.

5. Divide the mixture among the muffin cups, using a scant ⅓ cup for each.

6. Bake for 18 to 20 minutes or until the oatmeal is firm. Serve.

Diabetes Tip: To make this a diabetes-friendly recipe, substitute the brown sugar with 4 tablespoons powdered erythritol. The sugar content will decrease to 5 grams per serving.

Nutrition Info for 2 Oatmeal Cups: Calories: 296; Total fat: 10g; Saturated fat: 1g; Sodium: 84mg; Phosphorus: 236mg; Potassium: 289mg; Carbohydrates: 45g; Fiber: 6g; Protein: 8g; Sugar: 11g

Peanut Butter Bread Pudding Cups

LOW PROTEIN

Serves 6 • Prep time: 10 minutes • Cook time: 20 minutes

Bread pudding usually takes quite a bit of time. The bread cubes have to soak in custard, and the pudding itself bakes for about an hour. Using breadcrumbs instead of cubes takes away the soaking step, and using individual cups cuts the baking time to 20 minutes. These slightly sweet and savory cups are delicious served with some fresh fruit.

Baking spray

5 slices whole-wheat bread, coarsely crumbled

2 large eggs

½ cup unsweetened almond milk

¼ cup peanut butter

2 tablespoons honey

1 teaspoon vanilla

½ cup chopped unsalted peanuts

1. Preheat the oven to 375°F. Spray a 6-cup muffin tin with baking spray and set aside.

2. Put the breadcrumbs in a medium bowl.

3. In a small bowl, beat the eggs, milk, peanut butter, honey, and vanilla until smooth. Pour over the breadcrumbs.

4. Stir gently until combined, then divide the mixture evenly among the muffin cups. Sprinkle with the peanuts.

5. Bake for 18 to 20 minutes or until the puddings are set. Serve warm.

Make It Easier Tip: The fastest way to make breadcrumbs is to use a food processor or blender. Tear the bread into large pieces and place in the processor. Pulse until the bread forms similarly sized large crumbs.

Diabetes Tip: To make this a diabetes-friendly recipe, omit the honey and replace with 2 tablespoons and 2 teaspoons of powdered erythritol. The sugar content will decrease to 3 grams per serving.

Nutrition Info per Cup: Calories: 261; Total fat: 15g; Saturated fat: 3g; Sodium: 220mg; Phosphorus: 176mg; Potassium: 261mg; Carbohydrates: 24g; Fiber: 3g; Protein: 12g; Sugar: 9g

Warm Chia Pudding

HIGH FIBER, LOW PROTEIN

Serves 4 • Prep time: 10 minutes • Cook time: 5 minutes

Chia seeds may sound exotic, but they are available at most grocery stores. Chia seeds are a superfood and a great source of omega-3 fatty acids, antioxidants, and fiber. While the nutritional info appears to show that this pudding is high in phosphorus, remember that most of the phosphorus comes from the seeds and nuts, meaning that the phosphorus has low bioavailability and will be poorly absorbed in the body.

¾ cup chia seeds

3 cups unsweetened vanilla-flavored almond milk

3 tablespoons brown sugar

1 tablespoon unsalted butter

¼ teaspoon almond extract

¼ cup chopped unsalted pecans

½ cup plain whole-milk yogurt

1 cup sliced strawberries

1 cup blueberries

1. In a medium saucepan over medium heat, stir together the chia seeds, almond milk, brown sugar, and butter and bring to a simmer.

2. Reduce heat to medium-low and simmer, stirring frequently, until the pudding is thick, about 3 to 5 minutes.

3. Remove the pan from the heat and stir in the almond extract and pecans.

4. Serve, topped with the yogurt and berries.

Make It Easier Tip: You don't have to cook this pudding if you make it the night before. Just combine the chia seeds, almond milk, and substitute 1 tablespoon honey for the brown sugar. Put in a bowl and stir, then cover tightly. Refrigerate overnight. Then stir it in the morning, add the toppings, and enjoy!

Diabetes Tip: To make this a diabetes-friendly recipe, replace the 3 tablespoons of brown sugar with 4 tablespoons of powdered erythritol. The sugar content will decrease to 8 grams per serving.

Nutrition Info per Serving: Calories: 320; Total fat: 20g; Saturated fat: 4g; Sodium: 150 mg; Phosphorus: 339mg; Potassium: 415mg; Carbohydrates: 31g; Fiber: 13g; Protein: 8g; Sugar: 14g

Peanut Butter Granola

HIGH FIBER, LOW PROTEIN

Serves 4 • Prep time: 10 minutes • Cook time: 20 minutes

Homemade granola puts the packaged variety to shame. It's fresher, with more flavor and texture. Making your own means you can control the amount of sugar in it. You'll find yourself making this granola often because it's easy, satisfying, and uses ingredients you likely already have on hand.

2½ cups old-fashioned oats

½ cup coarsely chopped unsalted peanuts

⅓ cup peanut butter

2 tablespoons maple syrup

1 tablespoon peanut oil

2 teaspoons vanilla

1 teaspoon cinnamon

1. Preheat the oven to 350°F. Line a baking sheet or jelly roll pan with parchment paper or foil and set aside.

2. In a large bowl, mix together the oats and peanuts. Set aside.

3. In a small saucepan, over low heat, combine the peanut butter, maple syrup, and peanut oil. Heat, stirring, until the mixture is liquid and smooth, about 2 minutes.

4. Pour the peanut butter mixture over the granola and add the vanilla and cinnamon; mix well to coat.

5. Spread the granola mixture onto the baking sheet.

6. Bake for 15 to 20 minutes, stirring once, until the granola is toasted.

7. Cool on the baking sheet on a wire rack for 15 minutes, then break into pieces. Store the granola in an airtight container at room temperature for up to 4 days.

Increase Protein Tip: To make this a medium-protein recipe, increase the peanut butter to ½ cup, and add another ¼ cup of peanuts. The protein content will increase to 16 grams per serving.

Diabetes Tip: To make this a diabetes-friendly recipe, omit the maple syrup and increase the cinnamon to 2 teaspoons. The carbohydrate content will decrease to 23 grams, and the sugar content will drop to 4 grams.

Nutrition Info for a ¾ Cup Serving: Calories: 373; Total fat: 25g; Saturated fat: 5g; Sodium: 93mg; Phosphorus: 213mg; Potassium: 336mg; Carbohydrates: 30g; Fiber: 5g; Protein: 12g; Sugar: 10g

Savory Herb Waffles

DIABETES-FRIENDLY, LOW PROTEIN

Serves 6 • Prep time: 15 minutes • Cook time: 15 minutes

Waffles don't have to be a sweet meal. This savory version is a nice change of pace and works well served with some sautéed veggies or salsa if you like things spicy. These waffles can be made ahead of time, frozen, then reheated in a toaster right from the freezer until crisp and hot.

¾ cup all-purpose flour

¾ cup whole-wheat flour

½ cup yellow cornmeal

1½ teaspoons Low Phosphorus Baking Powder (page 140)

½ teaspoon dried thyme leaves

½ teaspoon dried basil leaves

Pinch salt

1½ cups plain whole-milk yogurt

¾ cup unsweetened almond milk

1 large egg, yolk and white separated

2 egg whites

2 tablespoons olive oil

1. In a medium bowl, whisk together the all-purpose flour, whole-wheat flour, corn-meal, baking powder, thyme, basil, and salt until well blended.

2. In a small bowl, combine the yogurt, almond milk, egg yolk, and olive oil.

3. In another small bowl, beat the egg whites with electric hand beaters until stiff peaks form, 2 to 3 minutes.

4. Stir the yogurt mixture into the flour mixture until just combined. Gently fold in the egg whites.

5. Heat a waffle iron according to manufacturer's instructions.

6. Add about ¼ cup of the batter to each section or fill according to the manufacturer's instructions.

7. Cook until the waffles stop steaming, about 4 to 5 minutes for each. Serve hot.

Increase Protein Tip: To make this a medium-protein recipe, serve each portion with 1 egg (any style). Adding an egg will increase the protein content of this meal to 15 grams per serving.

Tip: You can use this batter to make pancakes. Increase the almond milk to 1 cup. For sweet pancakes, omit the herbs and add 2 tablespoons sugar to the batter. Spoon the batter, using a ¼-cup measure, onto a greased skillet over medium heat. When the surface of the pancake bubbles and it looks crisp around the edges, about 2 to 3 minutes, flip them and cook for 1 to 2 minutes on the second side.

Nutrition Info for ⅙ Recipe: Calories: 246; Total fat: 9g; Saturated fat: 2g; Sodium: 189mg; Phosphorus: 171mg; Potassium: 319mg; Carbohydrates: 34g; Fiber: 3g; Protein: 9g; Sugar: 3g

Dutch Pancake with Cherry Apple Compote

HIGH FIBER, LOW PROTEIN

Serves 4 • Prep time: 5 minutes • Cook time: 25 minutes

A Dutch pancake is simply a large pancake that bakes in the oven instead of a skillet. The pancake rises in the oven, then falls as it cools, creating a space to add fruit or yogurt. This pancake recipe uses whole-wheat flour for fiber and is served with roasted cherries for a wonderful treat. You can fill this pancake with any type of fruit you'd like, such as sliced strawberries and blueberries.

1 tablespoon olive oil

1 tablespoon unsalted butter

¾ cup all-purpose flour

¾ cup whole-wheat flour

1 cup unsweetened almond milk

2 large eggs

2 egg whites

2 tablespoons brown sugar, divided

1 teaspoon vanilla

1 cup canned pitted sweet cherries in juice, drained

½ cup unsweetened applesauce

1. Preheat the oven to 400°F. Combine the olive oil and butter in an oven-safe skillet and set aside.

2. Combine the all-purpose flour, whole-wheat flour, milk, eggs, egg whites, 1 tablespoon brown sugar, and vanilla in a blender or food processor. Blend or process until the mixture is smooth.

3. Put the skillet in the oven until the butter has melted. Carefully remove from the oven and swirl to coat the pan in melted butter. Pour the batter in and immediately put the skillet back into the oven.

4. Bake for 21 to 25 minutes or until the pancake is puffed and golden brown.

5. While the pancake is baking, combine the cherries with the remaining brown sugar in a skillet over medium heat. Cook the cherries until the cherries are soft and have released some juice, about 4 to 5 minutes, stirring frequently. Stir in the applesauce and heat for another 2 minutes.

6. After the pancake is removed from the oven, it will fall. Fill the fallen pancake with the cherry mixture and serve.

Increase Protein Tip: To make this a medium-protein recipe, serve your pancake with ¼ cup of nonfat plain Greek yogurt. The protein content will increase to 17 grams per serving.

Diabetes Tip: To make this a diabetes-friendly recipe, make the following changes: In step 2, use 1 tablespoon plus 1 teaspoon of powdered erythritol instead of brown sugar. In step 5, omit the brown sugar entirely. The sugar content will decrease to 11 grams per serving.

Nutrition Info per Serving: Calories: 340; Total fat: 10g; Saturated fat: 3g; Sodium: 107mg; Phosphorus: 174mg; Potassium: 319mg; Carbohydrates: 52g; Fiber: 5g; Protein: 11g; Sugar: 16g

Berry Drop Scones

LOW PROTEIN

Serves 4 to 6 • Prep time: 12 minutes • Cook time: 18 minutes

Most scone recipes require rolling out dough and cutting it into rounds or triangles. This easier version is made like a drop biscuit. It's filled with sweet and nutritious berries for lots of flavor. Cream of tartar is found in the spice aisle; it combines with baking soda to make a phosphorus-free leavening agent.

1 cup whole-wheat flour
¾ cup all-purpose flour
⅓ cup quick oats
½ teaspoon baking soda
1 teaspoon cream
 of tartar

1 large egg
¾ cup raspberry yogurt
2 tablespoons
 avocado oil

2 tablespoons
 unsweetened
 almond milk
½ cup raspberries
½ cup blueberries

1. Preheat the oven to 400°F. Line a baking sheet with parchment paper and set aside.

2. In a medium bowl, stir together the whole-wheat flour, all-purpose flour, oats, baking soda, and cream of tartar.

3. In a small bowl, stir together the egg, yogurt, oil, and milk until well mixed.

4. Pour the liquid ingredients into the dry ingredients and mix just until combined. Fold in the raspberries and blueberries.

5. Drop the mixture by tablespoons 2 inches apart on the prepared baking sheet.

6. Bake for 16 to 18 minutes or until the scones are lightly browned. Serve warm.

Make It Easier Tip: Frozen berries are a convenient option if you don't have fresh berries on hand.

Nutrition Info for 2 Scones: Calories: 236; Total fat: 7g; Saturated fat: 1g; Sodium: 137mg; Phosphorus: 162mg; Potassium: 284mg; Carbohydrates: 36g; Fiber: 4g; Protein: 7g; Sugar: 5g

Avocado French Toast

DIABETES-FRIENDLY, HIGH FIBER, LOW PROTEIN

Serves 4 • Prep time: 15 minutes • Cook time: 10 minutes

You've probably heard of avocado toast. But have you ever made avocado French toast? This twist transforms the breakfast recipe into something special. Many people with CKD avoid avocados because of their potassium content, but that isn't necessary. Those with potassium restrictions can safely eat avocados as long as the portion size is kept under control, like in this recipe.

1 large egg

1 large egg white

½ cup unsweetened almond milk

½ teaspoon dried thyme leaves

4 slices whole-wheat bread

1 tablespoon unsalted butter

1 ripe avocado

1 tablespoon freshly squeezed lemon juice

2 scallions, white and green parts, chopped

1. In a shallow bowl, combine the egg, egg white, milk, and thyme leaves and beat until smooth.

2. Dip the bread slices into the egg mixture, turning once, letting the slices sit in the egg for 1 minute to absorb the custard.

3. In a large skillet, heat the butter over medium heat. Arrange the bread slices in a single layer in the skillet.

4. Cook for 3 to 5 minutes on each side, turning once until the bread is golden brown.

5. Meanwhile, in a small bowl, mash the avocado and lemon juice together with a fork. Stir in the scallions.

6. Serve the French toast topped with the avocado mixture.

Increase Protein Tip: To make this a medium-protein recipe, top the avocado French toast with one egg (any style). The protein content will increase to 15 grams per serving.

Nutrition Info per Serving: Calories: 205; Total fat: 11g; Saturated fat: 3g; Sodium: 219mg; Phosphorus: 124mg; Potassium: 332mg; Carbohydrates: 20g; Fiber: 5g; Protein: 8g; Sugar: 2g

Savory Turkey Frittata

DIABETES-FRIENDLY, MEDIUM PROTEIN

Serves 6 • Prep time: 14 minutes • Cook time: 16 minutes

A frittata is similar to an omelet, but it is finished in the oven and can be served hot or at room temperature. This recipe packs lots of flavor from heaps of onions, garlic, peppers, and basil. This satisfying egg dish is quick to make and will keep you full until it's time for lunch. You can even buy pre-chopped onions, garlic, and bell peppers to save more time.

1 tablespoon olive oil

12 ounces 93-percent-lean ground turkey

1 onion, diced

2 garlic cloves, minced

1 red bell pepper, cut into strips

8 large eggs

4 egg whites

1 teaspoon dried basil leaves

⅛ teaspoon freshly ground black pepper

¼ cup grated Parmesan cheese

1. In an ovenproof 8-inch skillet, heat the olive oil over medium heat. Add the turkey, onion, and garlic; cook and stir for 4 to 5 minutes. Add the bell pepper; cook and stir for 1 minute longer.

2. Meanwhile, beat the eggs, egg whites, basil, and pepper in a medium bowl until well combined.

3. Pour the eggs into the skillet.

4. Preheat the oven to broil and adjust the top rack so it is 6 inches from the heat.

5. Cook the eggs, stirring occasionally at first until the frittata begins to set, lifting the edges so the uncooked egg can flow underneath until the bottom is browned, but the top is still wet, about 8 minutes.

6. Transfer the skillet to the oven and broil for 2 to 3 minutes or until the top is lightly browned and the eggs are set. Top with the Parmesan, then cut into wedges to serve.

Increase Protein Tip: To make this a high-protein recipe, serve with 1 slice of whole-wheat toast. The protein content will increase to 25 grams per serving.

Nutrition Info per Serving: Calories: 216; Total fat: 13g; Saturated fat: 4g; Sodium: 186mg; Phosphorus: 228mg; Potassium: 282mg; Carbohydrates: 4g; Fiber: 1g; Protein: 21g; Sugar: 2g

Crustless Tex-Mex Quiche Cups

DIABETES-FRIENDLY, MEDIUM PROTEIN

Makes 12 cups • Prep time: 5 minutes • Cook time: 25 minutes

These little crustless quiches are simple to make. Their lack of crust helps reduce the refined carbohydrate content and cuts the preparation time by about 15 minutes. The addition of chili powder and cayenne pepper make these little cups spicy; you can add more of both spices if you'd like—or remove them entirely if you don't like spicy food.

Baking spray

2 tablespoons olive oil

1½ pounds 93-percent lean ground turkey

4 scallions, white and green parts, chopped

8 large eggs

2 teaspoons chili powder

⅛ teaspoon cayenne pepper

1 cup frozen corn, thawed

1 cup shredded cheddar cheese

1. Preheat the oven to 375°F. Spray a 12-cup muffin tin with baking spray and set aside.

2. In a medium skillet over medium heat, cook the ground turkey, stirring to break up the meat, for 5 to 7 minutes.

3. Add the scallions and cook for another 2 minutes or until the meat is cooked and the onions are tender. Remove from the heat and drain any excess oil.

4. In a medium bowl, beat the eggs, chili powder, and cayenne pepper.

5. Divide the meat mixture among the 12 muffin cups. Top with the corn.

6. Evenly divide the egg mixture between the muffin cups and top with the cheese.

7. Bake for 15 to 20 minutes or until the egg mixture is set. Cool for 3 minutes and serve.

Make It Easier Tip: This recipe works as a great make-ahead meal. Just bake, cool, cover, and put the muffins in the refrigerator. When ready to eat, micro-wave one muffin on high power for 15 seconds and enjoy.

Nutrition Info for 1 Quiche Cup: Calories: 210; Total fat: 14g; Saturated fat: 4g; Sodium: 156mg; Phosphorus: 224mg; Potassium: 226mg; Carbohydrates: 4g; Fiber: 1g; Protein: 18g; Sugar: 1g

Gremolata Scrambled Eggs

DIABETES-FRIENDLY, MEDIUM PROTEIN

Serves 4 • Prep time: 15 minutes • Cook time: 10 minutes

Gremolata is a fresh herb sauce from Italy that is made from garlic, lemon, and parsley. This recipe adds fragrant, fresh basil for even more flavor. Eggs, especially egg whites, are a great staple food for CKD because they are satisfying without contributing too much protein or phosphorus to the diet. And you can purchase egg whites in a carton!

1 lemon

½ cup chopped
   flat-leaf parsley

⅓ cup chopped
   fresh basil

1 tablespoon olive oil

4 large eggs

4 egg whites

2 tablespoons
   unsweetened
   almond milk

⅛ teaspoon salt

⅛ teaspoon freshly
   ground black pepper

1 tablespoon
   salted butter

4 slices whole-wheat
   toast, for serving

1. To make the gremolata, grate the zest from the lemon, then squeeze the juice, into a small bowl. Add the parsley, basil, and olive oil to the juice. Mix and set aside.

2. In a medium bowl, beat the eggs, egg whites, milk, salt, and pepper until smooth.

3. Heat a medium skillet over medium heat.

4. Add the butter and melt. Add the egg mixture to the skillet and drizzle half of the gremolata over the eggs.

5. Reduce the heat to medium-low and cook, stirring occasionally, until the eggs are scrambled and set, and cooked to 160°F (to kill Salmonella), about 8 to 10 minutes.

6. Drizzle the remaining gremolata over the eggs and serve with toast.

Reduce Protein Tip: For low protein, replace the whole-wheat toast with low-potassium fruit, such as ½ cup grapes. One serving of eggs plus the grapes would provide 11 grams of protein. If you're not restricting potassium, feel free to choose a higher potassium fruit, such as an orange.

Nutrition Info for 1 Serving Eggs + 1 Slice Whole-Wheat Toast: Calories: 250; Total fat: 12g; Saturated fat: 4g; Sodium: 388mg; Phosphorus: 178mg; Potassium: 288mg; Carbohydrates: 18g; Fiber: 3g; Protein: 15g; Sugar: 3g

Brie and Fruit Omelet

DIABETES-FRIENDLY, MEDIUM PROTEIN

Serves 4 • Prep time: 15 minutes • Cook time: 10 minutes

Omelets are often made with bacon and sausage, which contribute a lot of sodium and phosphorus to the dish. This recipe is deliciously different; the fruit adds a wonderful sweet taste, and the small amount of creamy Brie melts into the eggs beautifully. The combination is a perfect blend of savory and sweet.

2 tablespoons unsalted butter

1 peach, peeled, pitted, and cubed

1 pear, peeled, cored, and cubed

8 large eggs

½ teaspoon dried thyme leaves

½ cup diced Brie, rind removed

1. In an 8-inch skillet, melt the butter over medium heat.

2. Add the peach and pear cubes and sauté until they start to soften, 3 to 5 minutes. Remove the fruit from the skillet with a slotted spoon to a bowl and set aside.

3. In a medium bowl, beat the eggs and thyme until well blended. Pour the eggs into the skillet.

4. Cook the omelet over medium heat, stirring the eggs lightly at first and then lifting the edges to allow the uncooked egg to flow underneath. Continue cooking until the eggs are just set and the bottom is browned, about 5 to 6 minutes total.

5. Top the omelet evenly with the fruit and the Brie. Fold one half of the omelet over the other half and slide onto a platter. Serve immediately.

Increase Protein Tip: To make this a high-protein recipe, add 1 scoop (2 tablespoons) of an unflavored protein powder. Adding a protein powder with 30 grams protein per scoop will increase the recipe's protein content to 25 grams per serving.

Make It Easier Tip: Brie is easier to peel and dice when cold, so prepare it directly from the refrigerator. Remove the cheese from the refrigerator and peel it with a serrated knife and cut into tiny cubes. Don't refrigerate the diced Brie; if it's soft and warm, it will melt more easily into the omelet.

Nutrition Info per Serving: Calories: 306; Total fat: 22g; Saturated fat: 10g; Sodium: 239mg; Phosphorus: 221mg; Potassium: 279mg; Carbohydrates: 12g; Fiber: 2g; Protein: 17g; Sugar: 9g

Herbed Veggie Turkey Sausage

DIABETES-FRIENDLY, MEDIUM PROTEIN

Serves 6 • Prep time: 15 minutes • Cook time: 15 minutes

Once you make your own sausage, you might never buy premade again. This recipe is flavorful without being too high in sodium. You can cook this sausage right away or freeze it for later use. You can convert tasty sausages into a meal by topping one cooked patty with 2 tablespoons of Powerhouse Salsa (page 147), then wrapping it in one 6-inch corn tortilla.

2 teaspoons olive oil

1 medium onion, finely chopped

3 garlic cloves, minced

½ cup grated carrot

1 slice whole-wheat bread, crumbled

¾ pound 99-percent-lean ground turkey breast

1 large egg white

2 tablespoons chopped flat-leaf parsley

1 teaspoon dried thyme leaves

½ teaspoon dried sage leaves

⅛ teaspoon salt

⅛ teaspoon freshly ground black pepper

1. In a medium skillet, heat the olive oil over medium heat. Add the onion, garlic, and carrot and sauté for 3 to 4 minutes until tender.

2. Remove the vegetables to a large mixing bowl; stir in the breadcrumbs, and let stand 5 minutes.

3. Add the turkey, egg white, parsley, thyme, sage, salt, and pepper to the vegetables. Mix gently but thoroughly with your hands until combined.

4. Form the mixture into 6 patties, about ⅓-inch thick.

5. At this point, you can freeze the patties. Place each patty on a sheet of waxed paper, then put them into a freezer bag. Seal the bag, pressing out as much air as possible, mark with the date, and freeze.

6. To cook the sausage immediately, add the patties to the skillet over medium heat. Cook, turning once, about 5 to 6 minutes per side until the patties are browned and 165°F on a meat thermometer.

7. To cook from frozen, put the frozen patties into a skillet and turn the heat to medium. Cook, turning several times, about 8 to 9 minutes per side, until the patties are browned and a meat thermometer registers 165°F.

8. Serve with salsa in a tortilla.

Make It Easier Tip: Purchasing pre-grated carrots can save time. If you use this convenience product, cook the carrots 1 to 2 minutes longer to soften them because the pre-grated carrots are not as tender as freshly grated.

Nutrition Info per 1 Sausage Patty + 1 Corn Tortilla + 2 Tablespoons Powerhouse Salsa:
Calories: 179; Total fat: 4g; Saturated fat: 1g; Sodium: 155mg; Phosphorus: 264mg; Potassium: 428mg; Carbohydrates: 21g; Fiber: 3g; Protein: 18g; Sugar: 4g

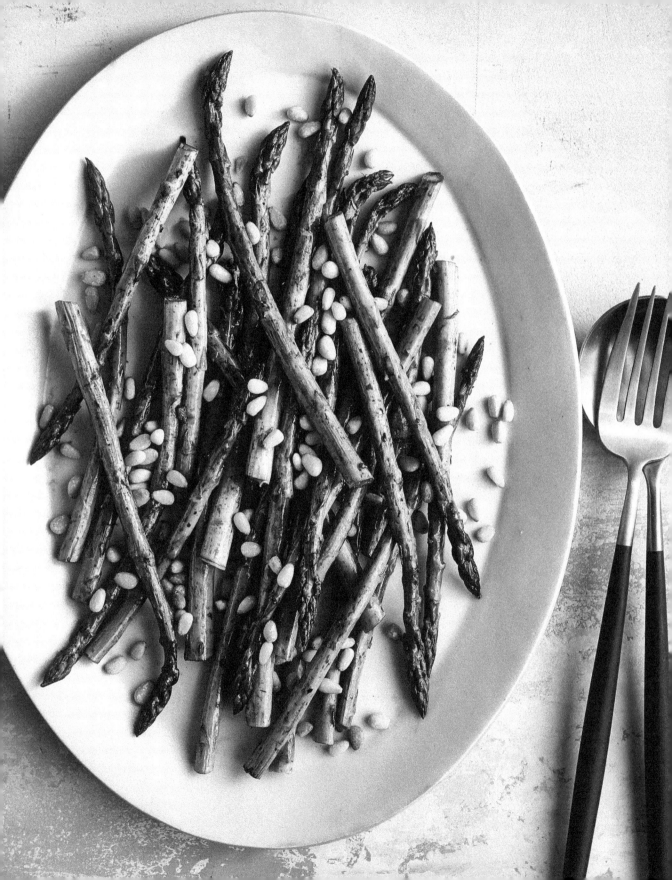

3

Vegetables, Sides, and Snacks

⇐ *Roasted Asparagus with Pine Nuts, page 44*

Roasted Broccoli and Cauliflower

DIABETES-FRIENDLY, HIGH FIBER, LOW PROTEIN, ONE POT

Serves 6 • Prep time: 7 minutes • Cook time: 23 minutes

Broccoli and cauliflower are two of the most nutrient-packed veggies you can eat. The lemon, Dijon mustard, and garlic powder add great flavor to this simple dish. Roasting these vegetables diminishes any bitterness and creates a delicious, tender texture. This easy side dish is excellent with grilled chicken or fish.

2 cups broccoli florets
2 cups cauliflower florets
2 tablespoons olive oil

1 tablespoon freshly squeezed lemon juice
2 teaspoons Dijon mustard

¼ teaspoon garlic powder
Pinch salt
⅛ teaspoon freshly ground black pepper

1. Preheat the oven to 425°F.
2. On a baking sheet with a lip, combine the broccoli and cauliflower florets in one even layer.
3. In a small bowl, combine the olive oil, lemon juice, mustard, garlic powder, salt, and pepper until well blended and drizzle the mixture over the vegetables. Toss to coat and spread the vegetables out in a single layer again.
4. Roast for 18 to 23 minutes or until the vegetables are brown around the edges and tender. Serve immediately.

Make It Easier Tip: To save time prepping, purchase fresh broccoli and cauliflower florets prepackaged (they are often combined together). Stick to fresh vegetables for this recipe because frozen vegetables won't roast well due to their high water content.

Nutrition Info per Serving: Calories: 63; Total fat: 5g; Saturated fat: 1g; Sodium: 74mg; Phosphorus: 39mg; Potassium: 216mg; Carbohydrates: 5g; Fiber: 2g; Protein: 2g; Sugar: 1g

Herbed Garlic Cauliflower Mash

DIABETES-FRIENDLY, HIGH FIBER, LOW PROTEIN

Serves 6 • Prep time: 20 minutes • Cook time: 10 minutes

Mashed cauliflower is a delicious alternative to mashed potatoes. Because cauliflower is much lower in carbohydrates and potassium than potatoes, this vegetable is an ideal choice for people with diabetes who are also restricting potassium. Cream cheese and herbs add flavor to this creamy, comforting dish.

4 cups cauliflower florets

4 garlic cloves, peeled

4 ounces cream cheese, softened

¼ cup unsweetened almond milk

2 tablespoons unsalted butter

Pinch salt

2 tablespoons minced fresh chives

2 tablespoons chopped flat-leaf parsley

1 tablespoon fresh thyme leaves

1. Bring a large pot of water to a boil over high heat. Add the cauliflower and garlic and cook, stirring occasionally, until the cauliflower is tender, about 8 to10 minutes.

2. Drain the cauliflower and garlic into a colander in the sink and shake the colander well to remove excess water.

3. Using a paper towel, blot the vegetables to remove any remaining water. Return the florets to the pot and place over low heat for 1 minute to remove as much water as possible.

4. Mash the florets and garlic with a potato masher until smooth.

5. Beat in the cream cheese, almond milk, butter, salt, chives, parsley, and thyme with a spoon. Serve.

Make It Easier Tip: Don't have any fresh herbs on hand? Dried herbs will work well, too. Replace every tablespoon of fresh herbs with 1 teaspoon of the dried variety.

Nutrition Info per Serving: Calories: 124; Total fat: 11g; Saturated fat: 6g; Sodium: 115mg; Phosphorus: 59mg; Potassium: 266mg; Carbohydrates: 6g; Fiber: 2g; Protein: 3g; Sugar: 2g

Sautéed Spicy Cabbage

DIABETES-FRIENDLY, HIGH FIBER, LOW PROTEIN

Serves 6 • Prep time: 15 minutes • Cook time: 5 minutes

If you have only eaten cabbage fresh in a salad, you will be surprised how delicious it is cooked. When sautéed with some garlic, it becomes tender and slightly sweet. Feel free to eliminate the cayenne pepper if you'd prefer a milder flavor—or use black or white pepper instead.

3 tablespoons olive oil

3 cups chopped
  green cabbage

3 cups chopped
  red cabbage

2 garlic cloves, minced

⅛ teaspoon
  cayenne pepper

Pinch salt

1. Heat the olive oil in a large skillet over medium heat.

2. Add the red and green cabbage and the garlic; sauté until the leaves wilt and are tender, about 4 to 5 minutes.

3. Sprinkle the vegetables with the cayenne pepper and salt, toss, and serve.

Make It Easier Tip: You can usually buy shredded cabbage that's intended for coleslaw in the produce aisle of the supermarket. Substitute it for the cabbage in this recipe to cut the prep time.

Nutrition Info per Serving: Calories: 86; Total fat: 7g; Saturated fat: 1g; Sodium: 46mg; Phosphorus: 27mg; Potassium: 189mg; Carbohydrates: 6g; Fiber: 2g; Protein: 1g; Sugar: 3g

Fragrant Thai-Style Eggplant

DIABETES-FRIENDLY, HIGH FIBER, LOW PROTEIN

Serves 6 • Prep time: 10 minutes • Cook time: 20 minutes

Fragrant ginger root, garlic, lime, and basil are common ingredients in Thai cuisine, and they add wonderful flavor to this delicious, high-fiber eggplant dish. If you aren't familiar with eggplant, take a chance and try this recipe. It is simple to prepare and appealing. Don't be surprised if you add it to your repertoire.

1 large eggplant, peeled and cut into ½-inch slices

¼ teaspoon salt

1 tablespoon extra-virgin olive oil

1 tablespoon peeled and grated fresh ginger root

1 garlic clove, minced

2 tablespoons freshly squeezed lime juice

1 tablespoon water

2 tablespoons chopped fresh basil

1. Preheat the oven to 400°F.

2. On a baking sheet with a lip, arrange the eggplant slices and sprinkle evenly with the salt. Drizzle with the olive oil.

3. Bake the eggplant for 10 minutes, then remove the baking sheet from the oven and turn the slices over. Return the baking sheet to the oven and bake for 10 to 15 minutes longer or until the eggplant is tender.

4. Meanwhile, stir together the ginger, garlic, lime juice, water, and basil in a small bowl until well mixed.

5. Place the eggplant on a serving plate and drizzle with the ginger mixture. Serve warm or cool.

Make It Easier Tip: If you don't have fresh ginger root on hand, you can use ¼ teaspoon of ground ginger in its place.

Nutrition Info per Serving: Calories: 52; Total fat: 2g; Saturated fat: 0g; Sodium: 101mg; Phosphorus: 30mg; Potassium: 280mg; Carbohydrates: 8g; Fiber: 4g; Protein: 1g; Sugar: 4g

Roasted Asparagus with Pine Nuts

DIABETES-FRIENDLY, HIGH FIBER, LOW PROTEIN

Serves 4 • Prep time: 10 minutes • Cook time: 15 minutes

Asparagus is delicious when roasted, and pine nuts add a crunchy texture and an extra nutritional boost to this dish. Fresh asparagus is widely available and best during the spring and summer months, but you can find it year-round for an extra expense. Don't substitute frozen or canned asparagus because the texture will be too soft after roasting.

1 pound fresh asparagus, woody ends removed

1 tablespoon olive oil

1 tablespoon balsamic vinegar

3 garlic cloves, minced

½ teaspoon dried thyme leaves

¼ cup pine nuts

1. Preheat the oven to 400°F.

2. Rinse the asparagus and arrange in a single layer on a baking sheet.

3. In a small bowl, stir together the olive oil, balsamic vinegar, garlic, and thyme until well mixed.

4. Drizzle the dressing over the asparagus and toss to coat.

5. Roast the asparagus for 10 minutes and remove the baking sheet from the oven.

6. Sprinkle the pine nuts over the asparagus and return the baking sheet to the oven. Roast for another 5 to 7 minutes or until the pine nuts are toasted and the asparagus is tender and light golden brown. Serve.

Make It Easier Tip: Purchasing pre-peeled garlic will save you time.

Nutrition Info per Serving: Calories: 116; Total fat: 9g; Saturated fat: 1g; Sodium: 4mg; Phosphorus: 112mg; Potassium: 294mg; Carbohydrates: 7g; Fiber: 3g; Protein: 4g; Sugar: 3g

Roasted Radishes

DIABETES-FRIENDLY, HIGH FIBER, LOW PROTEIN

Serves 6 • Prep time: 10 minutes • Cook time: 20 minutes

If you have never eaten roasted radishes before, you are in for a treat. This sharp and pungent root vegetable becomes tender and slightly sweet when roasted at a high temperature. If you need to restrict potassium or limit your carbohydrate intake, roasted radishes are a great substitute for roasted potatoes.

3 bunches whole
  small radishes

3 tablespoons olive
  oil, divided

1 tablespoon freshly
  squeezed lemon juice

1 tablespoon
  Dijon mustard

½ teaspoon dried
  marjoram leaves

⅛ teaspoon
  white pepper

Pinch salt

2 tablespoons chopped
  flat-leaf parsley

1. Preheat the oven to 425°F. Line a baking sheet with a lip with parchment paper and set aside.

2. Scrub the radishes, remove the stem and root, and cut each in half or thirds, depending on the size. The radishes should be similarly sized, so they cook evenly.

3. Toss the radishes and 1 tablespoon olive oil on the baking sheet to coat and arrange the radishes in a single layer.

4. Roast the radishes for 18 to 20 minutes or until they are slightly golden and tender, but still crisp on the outside.

5. While the radishes are roasting, whisk together the remaining 2 tablespoons of olive oil with the lemon juice, mustard, marjoram, pepper, and salt in a small bowl.

6. When the radishes are done, remove them from the baking sheet and place them in a serving bowl. Drizzle the vegetables with the dressing and toss. Sprinkle with the parsley. Serve warm or cool.

Make It Easier Tip: Reduce your prep time by roasting the radishes whole and increasing the cooking time to 25 minutes. When they are tender, drizzle with the dressing and serve.

Nutrition Info per Serving: Calories: 79; Total fat: 7g; Saturated fat: 1g; Sodium: 123mg; Phosphorus: 23mg; Potassium: 232mg; Carbohydrates: 4g; Fiber: 2g; Protein: 1g; Sugar: 2g

Mushroom Celery Salad

DIABETES-FRIENDLY, HIGH FIBER, LOW PROTEIN

Serves 6 • Prep time: 20 minutes

This nutrient-packed recipe works as a great accompaniment to many dishes, especially grilled chicken or fish. The celery adds a crunchy texture, and the vinegar gives the dish a zesty flavor. This salad is unusual because it doesn't have any leafy greens, but it is simple, delicious, and highly nutritious.

1 pound button mushrooms

5 celery stalks

2 scallions, white and green parts

3 tablespoons extra-virgin olive oil

2 tablespoons apple cider vinegar

2 tablespoons minced fresh basil leaves

1 tablespoon Dijon mustard

1 garlic clove, minced

1 teaspoon freeze-dried chives

Pinch salt

1. Rinse, dry, and thinly slice the mushrooms, celery, and scallions. Place all three in a serving bowl.

2. In a small bowl, whisk together the olive oil, vinegar, basil, mustard, garlic, chives, and salt until blended.

3. Pour the dressing over the vegetables and toss to coat. Serve.

Make It Easier Tip: To save prep time, purchase your mushrooms pre-sliced.

Nutrition Info per Serving: Calories: 87; Total fat: 7g; Saturated fat: 1g; Sodium: 91mg; Phosphorus: 79mg; Potassium: 347mg; Carbohydrates: 4g; Fiber: 2g; Protein: 3g; Sugar: 2g

Caraway Coleslaw

DIABETES-FRIENDLY, HIGH FIBER, LOW PROTEIN

Serves 4 • Prep time: 5 minutes

Coleslaw is a refreshing and simple salad to make, especially if you use the bags of pre-shredded, pre-washed coleslaw mix found in most produce departments. You can whip up a batch in minutes. The easy dressing used here is full of flavor and can be added to other recipes. Coleslaw tastes better when the flavors mellow, so double up the recipe and keep this salad for several days in the refrigerator.

1 (10-ounce) bag coleslaw mix

2 tablespoons extra-virgin olive oil

2 tablespoons apple cider vinegar

1 tablespoon yellow mustard

1 teaspoon honey

1 teaspoon caraway seeds

⅛ teaspoon freshly ground black pepper

1. Put the coleslaw mix in a large bowl. Don't wash the coleslaw.

2. In a small bowl, combine the olive oil, vinegar, mustard, honey, caraway seeds, and pepper, and whisk until blended.

3. Pour the dressing over the coleslaw mix and toss to coat. Serve immediately or cover and chill for a few hours before serving. Toss again before serving.

Make It Easier Tip: There are several different types of shredded cabbage in most grocery stores. Combine different types to make this recipe your own.

Nutrition Info per Serving: Calories: 88; Total fat: 7g; Saturated fat: 1g; Sodium: 55mg; Phosphorus: 26mg; Potassium: 140mg; Carbohydrates: 6g; Fiber: 2g; Protein: 1g; Sugar: 4g

Mixed Greens Veggie Tossed Salad

DIABETES-FRIENDLY, HIGH FIBER, LOW PROTEIN, ONE POT

Serves 4 • Prep time: 20 minutes

If you have CKD and are limiting potassium, you may have been told by your health provider to limit spinach in your diet due to its high potassium content. What many people don't realize is that raw baby spinach, unlike cooked spinach, is not high in potassium so can be safely consumed without worrying about potassium intake.

3 tablespoons extra-virgin olive oil

1 tablespoon balsamic vinegar

½ teaspoon dried marjoram leaves

1 garlic clove, minced

Pinch salt

Pinch white pepper

2 cups butter lettuce leaves

2 cups fresh baby spinach leaves

1 cup grated carrots

1 cucumber, peeled and sliced

2 celery stalks, sliced

1. In a large salad bowl, combine the olive oil, vinegar, marjoram, garlic, salt, and pepper, and whisk until combined.

2. Add the lettuce, spinach, carrots, cucumber, and celery and toss to coat. Serve.

Make It Easier Tip: To save time prepping, purchase boxed or bagged, pre-washed salad greens and grated carrots. Don't rewash the greens.

Nutrition Info per Serving: Calories: 124; Total fat: 10g; Saturated fat: 1g; Sodium: 70mg; Phosphorus: 46mg; Potassium: 377mg; Carbohydrates: 7g; Fiber: 2g; Protein: 2g; Sugar: 3g

Creamy Cucumber Salad

DIABETES-FRIENDLY, LOW PROTEIN

Serves 4 • Prep time: 20 minutes

This refreshing and simple salad is perfect for a side dish in the summer, or just about any time really. The creamy dressing is very versatile and works with most vegetables, so try it with green beans, red bell peppers, sliced summer squash, or even zucchini for a change of pace.

2 cucumbers, peeled, seeded, and thinly sliced

⅛ teaspoon salt

4 ounces cream cheese, softened

⅓ cup unsweetened almond milk

3 scallions, white and green parts, chopped

½ teaspoon dried dill weed

1. Put the cucumbers in a colander and sprinkle with the salt. Toss to coat and set aside in the sink while you make the dressing.

2. Put the cream cheese in a salad bowl and beat with electric hand beaters until smooth. Gradually add the almond milk until the mixture is creamy. Stir in the scallions and dill weed.

3. The cucumbers should have given up some liquid by now. Rinse them and drain, then blot with paper towels to remove the excess liquid.

4. Gently stir the cucumbers into the dressing. Serve immediately or chill for a few hours before serving.

Make It Easier Tip: If you can find English cucumbers, use them instead of the regular, fatter cucumbers. English cucumbers have tender skin, and their few seeds aren't bitter. Using English cucumbers will save you the task of peeling and deseeding the cucumbers before use.

Nutrition Info per Serving: Calories: 121; Total fat: 10g; Saturated fat: 6g; Sodium: 181mg; Phosphorus: 61mg; Potassium: 228mg; Carbohydrates: 6g; Fiber: 1g; Protein: 3g; Sugar: 3g

Two Bean Salad

Serves 4 • Prep time: 15 minutes • Cook time: 10 minutes

Green beans and yellow wax beans combine beautifully in this savory and slightly sweet salad. Using frozen green beans and canned wax beans keeps the prep time to a minimum. Red onion adds a slightly spicy note, and the lemon juice brightens this dish with its tart flavor. It will keep for three days in the refrigerator.

1 (10-ounce) package
   frozen green beans
1 (14-ounce) can wax
   beans, drained
   and rinsed

⅓ cup diced red onion
2 tablespoons olive oil
2 tablespoons freshly
   squeezed lemon juice
1 teaspoon honey

2 tablespoons chopped
   flat-leaf parsley

1. Cook the green beans as directed on the package and drain well.

2. Combine the green beans, wax beans, and red onion in a medium bowl.

3. In a small bowl, stir together the olive oil, lemon juice, and honey until blended.

4. Pour the dressing over the vegetables and toss to coat. Sprinkle with the parsley. Serve immediately or refrigerate for a few hours before serving.

Ingredient Tip: You can sometimes find frozen wax beans or canned low-sodium wax beans in your supermarket; use them instead of the regular canned wax beans for a lower sodium content. If you want to use fresh beans, steam them for 3 to 5 minutes over simmering water until tender.

Nutrition Info per Serving: Calories: 124; Total fat: 7g; Saturated fat: 1g; Sodium: 253mg; Phosphorus: 50mg; Potassium: 293mg; Carbohydrates: 14g; Fiber: 3g; Protein: 3g; Sugar: 5g

Grilled Peppers in Chipotle Vinaigrette

DIABETES-FRIENDLY, LOW PROTEIN

Serves 4 • Prep time: 15 minutes • Cook time: 6 minutes

Grilling vegetables intensifies their flavors and creates a delicious, difficult-to-resist silky texture. You can grill outside on a gas or charcoal grill, or inside on a grill pan or a two-sided grill if you prefer. This spicy vinaigrette adds another layer of flavor to the sweet bell peppers in this dish.

1 red bell pepper

1 yellow bell pepper

1 orange bell pepper

2 tablespoons extra-virgin olive oil

Juice of 1 lemon

1 teaspoon minced chipotle peppers in adobo sauce

1. Prepare and preheat the grill to medium coals and set a grill 6 inches from the coals. If grilling indoors, heat the grill pan over medium-high heat. For charcoal grills, medium coals mean you can hold your palm 6 inches above the grill rack for 3 to 4 seconds before you have to take it away. For gas and propane grills, medium coals are 350°F to 375°F.

2. Wash the bell peppers, remove the seeds, and cut them into 1-inch strips.

3. In a small bowl, stir together the olive oil, lemon juice, and chipotle peppers in adobo sauce.

4. Place the peppers on the grill and brush with some of the sauce. Grill the peppers for 2 to 3 minutes per side, brushing with the sauce occasionally, until the vegetables are tender and have defined grill marks. Serve.

Ingredient Tip: Chipotle peppers in adobo sauce are smoked jalapeños preserved in a spicy red sauce. Mince the peppers and measure out the sauce separately. This ingredient is readily available in the ethnic aisle of the supermarket.

Nutrition Info per Serving: Calories: 66; Total fat: 5g; Saturated fat: 1g; Sodium: 90mg; Phosphorus: 22mg; Potassium: 201mg; Carbohydrates: 6g; Fiber: 1g; Protein: 1g; Sugar: 5g

Double Corn Muffins

LOW PROTEIN

Makes 6 muffins • Prep time: 10 minutes • Cook time: 20 minutes

If you are a fan of traditional cornbread, these hearty muffins might become a new favorite. The golden cornmeal and whole corn kernels add lots of flavor and texture, and the brown sugar adds a hint of delectable sweetness. These muffins are perfect for an unusual side dish or a filling afternoon snack. You can reheat them in the microwave for 10 seconds per muffin and serve them warm with a little butter or plain.

¾ cup all-purpose flour
¼ cup yellow cornmeal
2 tablespoons brown sugar

1 teaspoon cream of tartar
½ teaspoon baking soda
Pinch salt
1 large egg

½ cup unsweetened almond milk
½ cup whole kernel corn
3 tablespoons unsalted butter, melted

1. Preheat the oven to 350°F. Line a 6-cup muffin pan with paper liners and set aside.

2. In a medium bowl, whisk together the flour, cornmeal, brown sugar, cream of tartar, baking soda, and salt until well blended.

3. In a small bowl, stir together the egg, milk, corn, and melted butter.

4. Add the liquid ingredients to the dry ingredients and stir just until combined. Don't overmix or the muffins will be tough.

5. Divide the batter among the prepared muffin cups, filling each about ¾ full.

6. Bake for 18 to 20 minutes or until the muffins are set and light golden brown.

7. Remove the muffins from the muffin tin and set on a wire rack to cool. Serve warm.

8. Store in a sealed container at room temperature for up to 3 days or freeze for up to 1 month.

Ingredient Tip: For this recipe, you can use thawed and drained frozen corn, fresh corn, or canned corn. If using canned corn, make sure to look for a low-sodium or no-salt-added product.

Nutrition Info per Muffin: Calories: 165; Total fat: 7g; Saturated fat: 4g; Sodium: 160mg; Phosphorus: 55mg; Potassium: 168mg; Carbohydrates: 22g; Fiber: 1g; Protein: 4g; Sugar: 3g

Creamy Carrot Hummus Dip

DIABETES-FRIENDLY, HIGH FIBER, LOW PROTEIN

Serves 6 • Prep time: 15 minutes

Hummus is a popular Middle Eastern dip and spread that is made with chickpeas, also called garbanzo beans. Just a few chickpeas along with carrots and garlic are used to make this delicious and colorful variation. Serve with Crisp Seeded Crackers (page 57) or fresh vegetables such as baby carrots, sliced zucchini, and celery sticks.

½ cup canned no-salt-added or low-sodium chickpeas, rinsed and drained

½ (14.5-ounce) can low-sodium carrots, rinsed and drained
2 garlic cloves, minced
3 tablespoons tahini

Juice of 1 lemon
2 tablespoons water
¼ teaspoon ground cumin
2 tablespoons olive oil

1. Combine the chickpeas, carrots, garlic, tahini, lemon juice, water, and cumin in a blender or food processor and blend until very smooth.

2. Place the hummus in a serving bowl and drizzle with the olive oil. Serve with crackers or raw vegetables, such as cucumbers, for dipping.

3. Store the hummus for up to 3 days in the refrigerator.

Ingredient Tip: Tahini is a paste made from sesame seeds. If you can't find it or are allergic to sesame seeds, you can use the same quantity of peanut or almond butter as a replacement.

Nutrition Info per Serving: Calories: 116; Total fat: 9g; Saturated fat: 1g; Sodium: 24mg; Phosphorus: 77mg; Potassium: 122mg; Carbohydrates: 7g; Fiber: 2g; Protein: 3g; Sugar: 2g

Roasted Red Pepper Dip

5-INGREDIENT, DIABETES-FRIENDLY, HIGH FIBER, LOW PROTEIN

Serves 4 • Prep time: 10 minutes

Jarred roasted red peppers are available in most grocery stores in the condiment section. Make sure you take a look at the nutrition label for a brand that is low-sodium. This creamy dip has tons of flavor and is ready in minutes. Try this dip with baby carrots or spread on whole-grain crackers or even a sandwich instead of butter.

1 (7-ounce) jar roasted red peppers, drained

4 ounces cream cheese, softened

2 tablespoons freshly squeezed lemon juice

2 scallions, white and green parts, chopped

⅛ teaspoon garlic powder

1. Combine the peppers, cream cheese, lemon juice, scallions, and garlic powder in a blender or food processor and blend or process until smooth or desired texture is reached.

2. Serve immediately or cover and chill up to 2 hours before serving.

3. This dip can be stored in the refrigerator for 2 to 3 days.

Ingredient Tip: It is very easy to roast your own peppers. Cut them in half, remove the stem and seeds, and put them skin side up on a baking sheet. Broil the peppers 6 inches from the heat for about 15 minutes or until the skins are blackened. Place them into a plastic bag to cool until the skins are loose and then peel the skins off. Don't rinse the peeled peppers because this dilutes the flavor.

Nutrition Info per 3-Tablespoon Serving: Calories: 124; Total fat: 10g; Saturated fat: 6g; Sodium: 197mg; Phosphorus: 43mg; Potassium: 155mg; Carbohydrates: 7g; Fiber: 2g; Protein: 2g; Sugar: 2g

Cheesy Rice–Stuffed Mushrooms

DIABETES-FRIENDLY, MEDIUM PROTEIN

Serves 6 • Prep time: 10 minutes • Cook time: 20 minutes

Stuffed mushrooms are a classic party appetizer that can also make a great light lunch or a snack. Large portobello mushrooms are available at most grocery stores, but if you can't find them, 18 smaller mushrooms can be used instead. To create deeper space for the filling, you can scrape out the dark mushroom gills on the inside of the cap before filling, but that's not essential.

6 (3-inch-diameter) portobello mushrooms

1 tablespoon olive oil

1 small red onion, diced

1 cup shredded part-skim mozzarella cheese

½ cup cooked brown rice

½ teaspoon dried oregano leaves

Pinch salt

Pinch freshly ground black pepper

1. Preheat the oven to 400°F.
2. Carefully remove and dice the mushroom stems. Place the mushroom heads gill side up on the baking sheet and set aside.
3. In a small skillet over medium heat, heat the olive oil.
4. Sauté the mushroom stems and onion until the vegetables are tender-crisp, 3 to 4 minutes.
5. Remove the skillet from the heat and stir in the cheese, rice, oregano, salt, and pepper until well mixed.
6. Spoon the rice mixture into the mushrooms and bake them for 15 to 20 minutes or until they are tender. Serve.

Ingredient Tip: Mushrooms are grown in soil, so don't worry about dirt that clings to them; just rinse it off.

Nutrition Info per Serving: Calories: 109; Total fat: 6g; Saturated fat: 3g; Sodium: 155mg; Phosphorus: 161mg; Potassium: 188mg; Carbohydrates: 8g; Fiber: 1g; Protein: 6g; Sugar: 2g

Double Onion Spread

Serves 6 • Prep time: 15 minutes • Cook time: 10 minutes

Onions are nutritional powerhouses. In addition to containing several antioxidants, raw onions are high in heart-protective sulfuric compounds. This simple and delicious spread is very versatile and so easy to make. Spread on a cracker or on some toast for a quick snack or a light lunch.

1 (8-ounce) package
cream cheese,
softened

3 tablespoons freshly
squeezed lemon juice

2 small red onions, diced

6 scallions, white and
green parts, sliced

1 teaspoon dried
thyme leaves

1. Combine the cream cheese and lemon juice in a medium bowl and beat until smooth and creamy with electric hand beaters.

2. Stir in the remaining ingredients. Serve immediately or cover and chill for a few hours before serving.

3. Store this spread for up to 3 days in the refrigerator.

Ingredient Tip: Red onions are sweeter than yellow or white onions. If the onion flavor is still too strong for you, you can cover the diced onions with water and add a pinch of sugar. Let stand for 5 minutes, then drain and use in the recipe.

Nutrition Info per Serving: Calories: 148; Total fat: 13g; Saturated fat: 8g; Sodium: 122mg; Phosphorus: 51mg; Potassium: 117mg; Carbohydrates: 6g; Fiber: 1g; Protein: 3g; Sugar: 3g

Crisp Seeded Crackers

DIABETES-FRIENDLY, LOW PROTEIN

Makes 24 crackers • Prep time: 10 minutes • Cook time: 20 minutes

Homemade crackers are another treat that will spoil you for the boxed variety. These little crackers are quick to make and pair perfectly with any of the dips and spreads in this book. Three kinds of seeds add lots of crunch and texture. If you don't like one of the seeds called for in this recipe, just omit them and add more of the other types.

1½ cups
   whole-wheat flour
2 tablespoons unsalted
   sunflower seeds
2 tablespoons
   sesame seeds

1 teaspoon
   caraway seeds
1 teaspoon cream
   of tartar
½ teaspoon baking soda
Pinch salt
¼ cup water

2 tablespoons olive oil
2 tablespoons unsalted
   butter, melted
2 tablespoons
   unsweetened
   almond milk

1. Preheat the oven to 400°F. Line a baking sheet with parchment paper.

2. In a medium bowl, combine the flour, sunflower seeds, sesame seeds, caraway seeds, cream of tartar, baking soda, and salt and mix well.

3. In a small bowl, stir together the water, oil, butter, and milk until well blended.

4. Add the wet ingredients to the dry ingredients and mix until a dough forms. You may need to add a bit more water depending on the consistency of the dough.

5. Roll the dough out onto the parchment paper. Using a sharp knife or a pizza cutter, cut the dough into 2-inch squares. Prick each square all over with a fork.

6. Bake the crackers for 15 to 20 minutes or until they are crisp and light golden brown. Remove from the baking sheet and let cool on a wire rack.

7. Store the crackers for 4 to 5 days in an airtight container at room temperature.

Ingredient Tip: You can use just about any combination of seeds you'd like in this recipe. Try chia seeds, flaxseed, pumpkin seeds, fennel seeds, or coriander seeds depending on your taste.

Nutrition Info per 2 Crackers: Calories: 107; Total fat: 6g; Saturated fat: 2g; Sodium: 68mg; Phosphorus: 75mg; Potassium: 117mg; Carbohydrates: 12g; Fiber: 1g; Protein: 3g; Sugar: 0g

Spicy Tex-Mex Popcorn

DIABETES-FRIENDLY, HIGH FIBER, LOW PROTEIN

Serves 6 • Prep time: 10 minutes • Cook time: 10 minutes

Popcorn is a healthy snack, as long as it's air-popped and not slathered with excess butter and salt. In addition to being a good source of fiber, popcorn is delicious and fun to eat. Make this recipe for a party, or to snack on when you're watching a good movie.

12 cups air-popped popcorn (6 tablespoons unpopped)

3 tablespoons unsalted butter, melted

1 tablespoon chili powder

1 teaspoon ground cumin

1 teaspoon paprika

½ teaspoon dried oregano leaves

¼ teaspoon garlic powder

⅛ teaspoon onion powder

⅛ teaspoon salt

⅛ teaspoon cayenne pepper

1. Pour the popped corn into a large bowl.

2. Drizzle with the butter and toss.

3. In a small bowl, stir together the chili powder, cumin, paprika, oregano, garlic powder, onion powder, salt, and cayenne pepper until well blended.

4. Sprinkle the popcorn with the spice mixture and toss to coat. Serve.

Ingredient Tip: There are several methods you can use to pop your popcorn. You can air pop using a popcorn popper, or you can use a heavy saucepan on the stovetop. For the stovetop method, preheat a large empty covered pot on medium-high heat for 2 minutes. Add the popcorn kernels, cover, and immediately reduce the heat to low. Let the popcorn pop, gently shaking the covered pan frequently, until the popping slows to 1 to 2 pops every 3 seconds. This should take 5 to 6 minutes. Pour the popcorn into the bowl and proceed with the recipe.

Nutrition Info per 2 Cups: Calories: 120; Total fat: 7g; Saturated fat: 4g; Sodium: 90mg; Phosphorus: 67mg; Potassium: 99mg; Carbohydrates: 14g; Fiber: 3g; Protein: 2g; Sugar: 0g

Baby Carrot Fries

DIABETES-FRIENDLY, HIGH FIBER, LOW PROTEIN

Serves 6 • Prep time: 10 minutes • Cook time: 20 minutes

Carrot fries are a nutritious alternative to French fries. Packaged baby carrots are simply large carrots that have been trimmed down mechanically to a uniform size. Using baby carrots saves the step of peeling and cutting larger carrots into small pieces. You can find real baby carrots in the grocery store if you want a lovely sweet taste, but they are expensive and only available in the summer and early fall in most regions.

Cooking spray

1 large egg

2 tablespoons Dijon mustard

1 tablespoon freshly squeezed lemon juice

1 cup panko breadcrumbs

1 (16-ounce) package baby carrots, cut in half lengthwise

1. Preheat the oven to 425°F. Spray a rack that fits into a jelly roll pan with cooking spray and set aside.

2. In a shallow bowl, beat the egg, mustard, and lemon juice. Put the breadcrumbs on a plate.

3. Add the baby carrots to the egg mixture, tossing to coat.

4. Using a slotted spoon, transfer the carrots from the egg mixture to the breadcrumbs in batches and toss to coat the vegetables.

5. Transfer the breaded carrots to the rack on the prepared jelly roll pan and arrange the veggies in a single layer. Repeat until all the carrots are breaded.

6. Bake the carrot fries for 18 to 20 minutes or until the fries are tender and crispy. Serve.

Ingredient Tip: Most boxed panko breadcrumbs are low in sodium. Look for a brand with no more than 100 milligrams of sodium per serving. As always, check the ingredients to make sure there are no phosphate additives.

Nutrition Info per Serving: Calories: 145; Total fat: 6g; Saturated fat: 1g; Sodium: 217mg; Phosphorus: 61mg; Potassium: 233mg; Carbohydrates: 19g; Fiber: 4g; Protein: 3g; Sugar: 5g

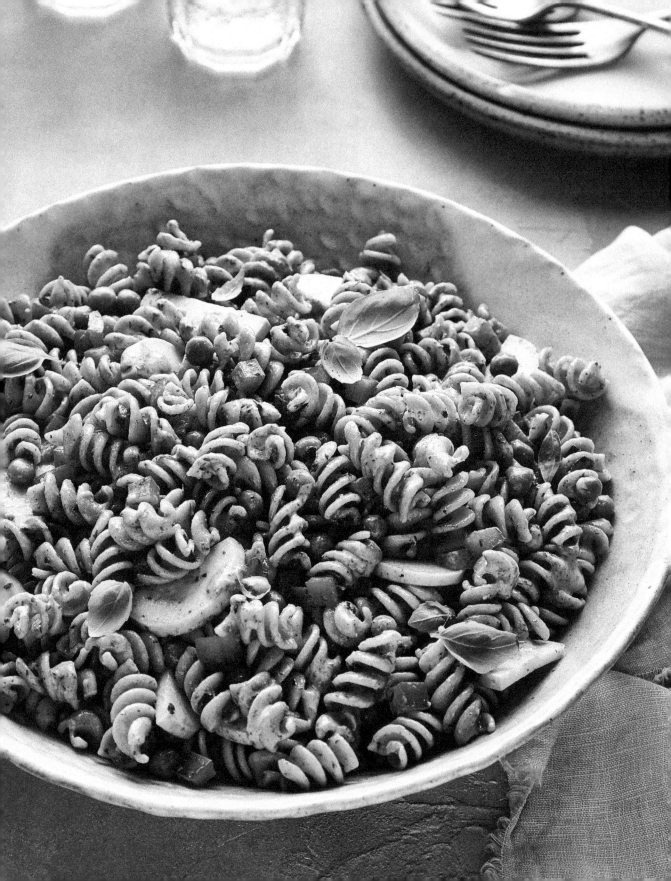

Vegetarian and Vegan Entrées

⇦ *Pesto Pasta Salad, page 67*

Curried Veggies and Rice

DIABETES-FRIENDLY, LOW PROTEIN, ONE POT

Serves 4 • Prep time: 12 minutes • Cook time: 18 minutes

Curry powder adds wonderful flavor and color to this easy recipe. Curry powder contains turmeric, a spice with significant anti-inflammatory potential. This simple stir-fry recipe is quick to make and is a satisfying dinner served with some fresh fruit.

¼ cup olive oil

1 cup long-grain white basmati rice

4 garlic cloves, minced

2½ teaspoons curry powder

½ cup sliced shiitake mushrooms

1 red bell pepper, chopped

1 cup frozen, shelled edamame

2 cups low-sodium vegetable broth

⅛ teaspoon freshly ground black pepper

1. Heat the olive oil in a large saucepan over medium heat.

2. Add the rice, garlic, curry powder, mushrooms, bell pepper, and edamame; cook, stirring, for 2 minutes.

3. Add the broth and black pepper and bring to a boil.

4. Reduce the heat to low, partially cover the pot, and simmer for 15 to 18 minutes or until the rice is tender. Stir and serve.

Increase Protein Tip: To make this a medium-protein recipe, beat 4 eggs, and add them to the rice mixture. Let stand for 3 to 4 minutes until the eggs are cooked and set, then stir to mix the eggs through the rice. The protein content will increase to 15 grams per serving.

Nutrition Info per Serving: Calories: 347; Total fat: 16g; Saturated fat: 2g; Sodium: 114mg; Phosphorus: 131mg; Potassium: 334mg; Carbohydrates: 44g; Fiber: 4g; Protein: 8g; Sugar: 3g

Spicy Mushroom Stir-Fry

DIABETES-FRIENDLY, LOW PROTEIN, ONE POT

Serves 4 • Prep time: 15 minutes • Cook time: 10 minutes

Stir-fry recipes are speedy to cook, but preparation time can be lengthy because the vegetables need different cooking times or need to be cut to a similar size. Purchasing pre-sliced mushrooms helps cut that time down. For those new to vegetarian meals, the meaty texture of mushrooms can help make up for the absence of meat.

1 cup low-sodium
 vegetable broth

2 tablespoons cornstarch

1 teaspoon low-sodium
 soy sauce

½ teaspoon
 ground ginger

⅛ teaspoon
 cayenne pepper

2 tablespoons olive oil

2 (8-ounce)
 packages sliced
 button mushrooms

1 red bell
 pepper, chopped

1 jalapeño pepper,
 minced

3 cups brown rice that
 has been cooked in
 unsalted water

2 tablespoons sesame oil

1. In a small bowl, whisk together the broth, cornstarch, soy sauce, ginger, and cayenne pepper and set aside.

2. Heat the olive oil in a wok or heavy skillet over high heat.

3. Add the mushrooms and peppers and stir-fry for 3 to 5 minutes or until the vegetables are tender-crisp.

4. Stir the broth mixture and add it to the wok; stir-fry for 3 to 5 minutes longer or until the vegetables are tender and the sauce has thickened. Serve the stir-fry over the hot cooked brown rice and drizzle with the sesame oil.

Ingredient Tip: If you don't like spicy food, feel free to omit or reduce the amount of jalapeño pepper and cayenne pepper used in this recipe.

Nutrition Info per Serving: Calories: 361; Total fat: 16g; Saturated fat: 2g; Sodium: 95mg; Phosphorus: 267mg; Potassium: 582mg; Carbohydrates: 49g; Fiber: 4g; Protein: 8g; Sugar: 4g

Spicy Veggie Pancakes

DIABETES-FRIENDLY, HIGH FIBER, LOW PROTEIN

Serves 4 • Prep time: 20 minutes • Cook time: 10 minutes

Homemade pancakes are a real treat. This unusual savory version is full of flavor and color from the grated carrot. Cayenne pepper and minced jalapeño peppers add zing to this easy vegetarian main dish. Serve with a generous scoop of Powerhouse Salsa (page 147) for a flavorful lunch or dinner.

3 tablespoons olive oil, divided

2 small onions, finely chopped

1 jalapeño pepper, minced

¾ cup carrot, grated

¾ cup cabbage, finely chopped

1½ cups quick-cooking oats

¾ cup cooked brown rice

¾ cup water

½ cup whole-wheat flour

1 large egg

1 large egg white

1 teaspoon baking soda

¼ teaspoon cayenne pepper

1. Heat 2 teaspoons oil in a medium skillet over medium heat.

2. Sauté the onion, jalapeño, carrot, and cabbage for 4 minutes.

3. While the veggies are cooking, combine the oats, rice, water, flour, egg, egg white, baking soda, and cayenne pepper in a medium bowl until well mixed.

4. Add the cooked vegetables to the mixture and stir to combine.

5. Heat the remaining oil in a large skillet over medium heat.

6. Drop the mixture into the skillet, about ⅓ cup per pancake. Cook for 4 minutes, or until bubbles form on the surface of the pancakes and the edges look cooked, then carefully flip them over.

7. Cook the second sides for 3 to 5 minutes or until the pancakes are hot and firm.

8. Repeat with the remaining mixture and serve.

Make It Easier Tip: To save on prep time, purchase pre-grated carrots and cabbage. Brown rice can also be bought frozen and then microwaved according to package directions when you're ready to use it.

Nutrition Info per Serving: Calories: 323; Total fat 11g; Saturated fat: 2g; Sodium: 366mg; Potassium: 381mg; Phosphorus: 263mg; Carbohydrates: 48g; Fiber: 7g; Protein: 10g; Sugar: 4g

Egg and Veggie Fajitas

DIABETES-FRIENDLY, HIGH FIBER, LOW PROTEIN

Serves 4 • Prep time: 20 minutes • Cook time: 10 minutes

The word fajita *means beef strips, but fajitas don't have to contain meat; any filling can be used. This savory and spicy mixture of eggs and vegetables is served tucked into a soft corn tortilla. This recipe makes an excellent meal no matter what time of day. You can make this dish spicier by adding another jalapeño pepper.*

3 large eggs

3 egg whites

2 teaspoons chili powder

1 tablespoon
   unsalted butter

1 onion, chopped

2 garlic cloves, minced

1 jalapeño pepper,
   minced

1 red bell
   pepper, chopped

1 cup frozen corn,
   thawed and drained

8 (6-inch) corn tortillas

1. Whisk the eggs, egg whites, and chili powder in a small bowl until well combined. Set aside.

2. In a large skillet, melt the butter over medium heat.

3. Sauté the onion, garlic, jalapeño, bell pepper, and corn, until the vegetables are tender, 3 to 4 minutes.

4. Add the beaten egg mixture to the skillet. Cook, stirring occasionally, until the eggs form large curds and are set, 3 to 5 minutes.

5. Meanwhile, soften the corn tortillas as directed on the package.

6. Divide the egg mixture evenly among the softened corn tortillas. Roll the tortillas up and serve.

Increase Protein Tip: To make this a medium-protein recipe, increase the egg whites to 6 and replace 1 cup frozen corn with 1 cup canned no-salt-added or low-sodium canned black beans. The protein will increase to 19 grams per serving.

Nutrition Info per Serving: Calories: 316; Total fat 14g; Saturated fat: 3g; Sodium: 167mg; Potassium: 408mg; Phosphorus: 287mg; Carbohydrates: 35g; Fiber: 5g; Protein: 14g; Sugar: 4g

Vegetable Biryani

DIABETES-FRIENDLY, HIGH FIBER, LOW PROTEIN, ONE POT

Serves 4 • Prep time: 20 minutes • Cook time: 10 minutes

Biryani is an Indian dish made of rice and vegetables that are spiced with curry powder. If you are new to curry powder, try several brands and add the one you like best. Curry powder can be mild or fiery hot depending on the ingredients used in the blend. This recipe is simple to make and can be bulked up by stuffing the rice mixture into a pita.

2 tablespoons olive oil

1 onion, diced

4 garlic cloves, minced

1 tablespoon peeled and grated fresh ginger root

1 cup carrot, grated

2 cups chopped cauliflower

1 cup frozen baby peas, thawed and drained

2 teaspoons curry powder

1 cup low-sodium vegetable broth

3 cups frozen cooked brown rice

1. In a large skillet, heat the olive oil over medium heat.
2. Add the onion, garlic, and ginger root and sauté, stirring frequently, until tender-crisp, 2 minutes.
3. Add the carrot, cauliflower, peas, and curry powder and cook for 2 minutes longer.
4. Stir in the vegetable broth and bring to a simmer. Reduce the heat to low, partially cover the skillet, and simmer for 6 to 7 minutes or until the vegetables are tender.
5. Meanwhile, heat the rice as directed on the package.
6. Stir the rice into the vegetable mixture and serve.

Nutrition Info per Serving: Calories: 378; Total fat 16g; Saturated fat: 2g; Sodium: 113mg; Potassium: 510mg; Phosphorus: 236mg; Carbohydrates: 53g; Fiber: 7g; Protein: 8g; Sugar: 6g

Pesto Pasta Salad

DIABETES-FRIENDLY, HIGH FIBER, LOW PROTEIN

Serves 4 • Prep time: 15 minutes • Cook time: 15 minutes

Pesto is a classic Italian green sauce that is typically made with at least one cup of oil, but this sauce doesn't need a lot of oil to be delicious. You can cut the oil and increase the vegetables with stellar results. The herbs in this recipe enhance the flavor, and the combination of vegetables lends brilliant color to the dish. Serve this salad warm or chilled.

1 cup fresh basil leaves

½ cup packed fresh flat-leaf parsley leaves

½ cup arugula, chopped

2 tablespoons Parmesan cheese, grated

¼ cup extra-virgin olive oil

3 tablespoons mayonnaise

2 tablespoons water

12 ounces whole-wheat rotini pasta

1 red bell pepper, chopped

1 medium yellow summer squash, sliced

1 cup frozen baby peas thawed and drained

1. Bring a large pot of water to boil.

2. Meanwhile, combine the basil, parsley, arugula, cheese, and olive oil in a blender or food processor. Blend or process until the herbs are finely chopped. Add the mayonnaise and water, then process again. Set aside.

3. Add the pasta to the pot of boiling water; cook according to package directions, about 8 to 9 minutes. Drain well, reserving ¼ cup of the cooking liquid.

4. Combine the pesto, pasta, bell pepper, squash, and peas in a large bowl and toss gently, adding enough of the reserved pasta cooking liquid to make a sauce on the salad. Serve immediately or cover and chill, then serve.

5. Store covered in the refrigerator up to 3 days.

Ingredient Tip: Since you don't cook the extra-virgin olive oil in this recipe, a good quality brand will contribute increased flavor and richness. Reserve the more expensive, higher quality extra-virgin olive oil for recipes like this one and stick to using regular olive oil for sautéing.

Nutrition Info per Serving: Calories: 378; Total fat 24g; Saturated fat: 4g; Sodium: 163mg; Potassium: 472mg; Phosphorus: 213mg; Carbohydrates: 35; Fiber: 6g; Protein: 9g; Sugar: 5g

Barley Blueberry Avocado Salad

DIABETES-FRIENDLY, HIGH FIBER, LOW PROTEIN

Serves 4 • Prep time: 15 minutes • Cook time: 15 minutes

This unusual and beautiful salad is delicious and full of wonderful flavors, textures, and colors. It is served warm, but you can chill it in the refrigerator for a couple of hours to serve cold. If you choose to chill it first, add the avocado just before serving, so it doesn't oxidize.

1 cup quick-cooking barley

3 cups low-sodium vegetable broth

3 tablespoons extra-virgin olive oil

2 tablespoons freshly squeezed lemon juice

1 teaspoon yellow mustard

1 teaspoon honey

½ avocado, peeled and chopped

2 cups blueberries

¼ cup crumbled feta cheese

1. In a medium saucepan, combine the barley and vegetable broth and bring to a simmer.

2. Reduce the heat to low, partially cover the pan, and simmer for 10 to 12 minutes or until the barley is tender.

3. Meanwhile, whisk together the olive oil, lemon juice, mustard, and honey in a serving bowl until blended.

4. Drain the barley if necessary and add to the bowl; toss to combine.

5. Add the avocado, blueberries, and feta and toss gently. Serve.

Increase Protein Tip: To make this a medium-protein recipe, omit the avocado and add 2 cups of thawed frozen edamame. The protein will increase to 16 grams per serving. Eliminating the avocado can also control the potassium content of the recipe. If you aren't restricting potassium, feel free to leave it in.

Nutrition Info per Serving: Calories: 345; Total fat 16g; Saturated fat: 3g; Sodium: 259mg; Potassium: 301mg; Phosphorus: 152mg; Carbohydrates: 44g; Fiber: 7g; Protein: 7g; Sugar: 11g

Pasta with Creamy Broccoli Sauce

DIABETES-FRIENDLY, HIGH FIBER, LOW PROTEIN

Serves 4 • Prep time: 15 minutes • Cook time: 15 minutes

When puréed with a little cream cheese, garlic, and some reserved pasta water, broccoli makes an elegant and silky sauce. This simple but indulgent recipe is perfect with whole-wheat pasta and a sprinkle of Parmesan cheese.

2 tablespoons olive oil
1 pound broccoli florets
3 garlic cloves, halved
1 cup low-sodium
  vegetable broth

½ pound whole-wheat
  spaghetti pasta
4 ounces cream cheese
1 teaspoon dried
  basil leaves

½ cup grated
  Parmesan cheese

1. Bring a large pot of water to a boil.

2. Meanwhile, heat a large skillet over medium heat and add the olive oil. Sauté the broccoli and garlic, stirring frequently, for 3 minutes.

3. Add the broth to the skillet and bring to a simmer. Reduce the heat to low, partially cover the skillet, and simmer until the broccoli is tender, about 5 to 6 minutes.

4. Cook the pasta according to package directions. Drain when al dente, reserving 1 cup pasta water.

5. When the broccoli is tender, add the cream cheese and basil. Purée using an immersion blender. You could also spoon the mixture into a blender or food processor, about half at a time, and purée until smooth, and transfer the sauce back into the skillet.

6. Add the cooked pasta to the broccoli sauce. Toss, adding enough pasta water until the sauce coats the pasta completely. Sprinkle with the Parmesan and serve.

Make It Easier Tip: Frozen broccoli can replace fresh broccoli in this recipe to save some time. Skip the sauté step and just simmer the broccoli with the garlic and the broth until it is tender.

Nutrition Info per Serving: Calories: 302; Total fat 14g; Saturated fat: 6g; Sodium: 260mg; Potassium: 375mg; Phosphorus: 223mg; Carbohydrates: 36g; Fiber: 5g; Protein: 11g; Sugar: 2g

Asparagus Fried Rice

DIABETES-FRIENDLY, LOW PROTEIN

Serves 4 • Prep time: 20 minutes • Cook time: 10 minutes

Fried rice is a classic Asian dish that works best when it is made with cold cooked rice. While you can certainly cook your own rice and cool it overnight before using, frozen rice is an easy substitution. Compared to restaurant-prepared fried rice, this recipe uses less soy sauce, making it a much lower sodium option.

3 large eggs, beaten

½ teaspoon ground ginger

2 teaspoons low-sodium soy sauce

2 tablespoons olive oil

1 onion, diced

4 garlic cloves, minced

1 cup sliced cremini mushrooms

1 (10-ounce) package frozen brown rice, thawed

8 ounces fresh asparagus, about 15 spears, cut into 1-inch pieces

1 teaspoon sesame oil

1. Whisk the eggs, ginger, and soy sauce in a small bowl and set aside.
2. Heat the olive oil in a medium skillet or wok over medium heat.
3. Add the onion and garlic and sauté for 2 minutes until tender-crisp.
4. Add the mushrooms and rice; stir-fry for 3 minutes longer.
5. Add the asparagus and stir-fry for 2 minutes.
6. Move the rice mixture to one side of the skillet and pour in the egg mixture. Stir the eggs until cooked through, 2 to 3 minutes, and stir into the rice mixture.
7. Sprinkle the fried rice with the sesame oil and serve.

Increase Protein Tip: To make this a medium-protein recipe, add 2 additional eggs, and in step 2, add 2 cups of frozen peas, as well. The protein content will increase to 16 grams per serving.

Nutrition Info per Serving: Calories: 247; Total fat 13g; Saturated fat: 3g; Sodium: 149mg; Potassium: 367mg; Phosphorus: 206mg; Carbohydrates: 25g; Fiber: 3g; Protein: 9g; Sugar: 3g

Tex-Mex Pepper Stir-Fry

DIABETES-FRIENDLY, HIGH FIBER, LOW PROTEIN

Serves 4 • Prep time: 20 minutes • Cook time: 10 minutes

Tex-Mex foods are packed with flavor and can be very nutritious. Black beans give this vegetarian stir-fry recipe a boost in fiber and are a delicious substitute for meat. This colorful recipe is spicy with garlic and jalapeño peppers. If you enjoy your food with even more heat, add ⅛ teaspoon cayenne pepper with the beans.

2 tablespoons olive oil

1 onion, chopped

4 garlic cloves, minced

1 jalapeño pepper, minced

1 red bell pepper, chopped

1 yellow bell pepper, chopped

1 cup canned no-salt-added or low-sodium black beans, rinsed and drained

½ cup Powerhouse Salsa (page 147)

Juice from 1 lemon

2 cups cooked brown rice

1. Heat the oil in a large wok or skillet over medium-high heat.

2. Add the onion and garlic and stir-fry for 2 minutes.

3. Stir in the jalapeño pepper, red bell pepper, and yellow bell pepper, and stir-fry for another 3 minutes.

4. Add the black beans and stir-fry for 3 to 5 minutes longer or until the ingredients are heated through.

5. Stir in the salsa and lemon juice and serve over the rice.

Make It Easier Tip: Frozen mixed red bell peppers are available in most supermarkets, so you can use 2 cups of this product instead of fresh pepper to save prep time.

Nutrition Info per Serving: Calories: 297; Total fat 8g; Saturated fat: 1g; Sodium: 29mg; Potassium: 589mg; Phosphorus: 212mg; Carbohydrates: 49g; Fiber: 9g; Protein: 8g; Sugar: 7g

Vegetarian Taco Salad

DIABETES-FRIENDLY, HIGH FIBER, LOW PROTEIN, ONE POT

Serves 4 • Prep time: 20 minutes

Taco salad is a colorful meal that can be ready in just a few minutes. Most taco salads contain seasoned beef, but not this one. Beans and rice substitute for the meat in this no-cook recipe and the plentiful vegetables add flavor and freshness. Keep these ingredients on hand so you can make this salad often, especially on hot summer days.

1½ cups canned low-sodium or no-salt-added pinto beans, rinsed and drained

1 (10-ounce) package frozen brown rice, thawed

1 red bell pepper, chopped

3 scallions, white and green parts, chopped

1 jalapeño pepper, minced

1 cup frozen corn, thawed and drained

1 tablespoon chili powder

1 cup chopped romaine lettuce

2 cups chopped butter lettuce

½ cup Powerhouse Salsa (page 147)

½ cup grated pepper Jack cheese

1. In a medium bowl, combine the beans, rice, bell pepper, scallions, jalapeño, and corn.

2. Sprinkle with the chili powder and stir gently. Stir in the romaine and butter lettuce.

3. Serve topped with Powerhouse Salsa and cheese.

Increase Protein Tip: To make this a medium-protein recipe, serve each portion with 1 egg (any style). The protein content will increase to 18 grams.

Nutrition Info per Serving: Calories: 254; Total fat 7g; Saturated fat: 3g; Sodium: 440mg; Potassium: 599mg; Phosphorus: 240mg; Carbohydrates: 39g; Fiber: 8g; Protein: 11g; Sugar: 5g

Creamy Red Pepper Pasta

DIABETES-FRIENDLY, HIGH FIBER, LOW PROTEIN

Serves 6 • Prep time: 15 minutes • Cook time: 15 minutes

When you have CKD and need to limit potassium, tomato sauce is usually on the do-not-eat list. Due to their lower potassium content, red peppers are wonderful as a substitute for tomatoes in this tasty and comforting recipe. Make sure that the peppers cook until they are very tender, so they purée into a velvety sauce.

2 tablespoons olive oil

1 leek, white and green parts, cleaned and chopped

2 garlic cloves, minced

2 large red bell peppers, thinly sliced

1 cup low-sodium vegetable broth

12 ounces whole-wheat fettuccine pasta

1 (8-ounce) package cream cheese, softened

1 teaspoon dried marjoram leaves

2 tablespoons grated Parmesan cheese

1. Bring a large pot of water to a boil.

2. Meanwhile, heat the olive oil over medium heat in a large skillet.

3. Add the leek, garlic, and bell peppers; sauté for 3 to 4 minutes or until tender.

4. Stir in the broth and simmer for 2 minutes.

5. Add the pasta to the boiling water and cook until al dente according to package directions. Drain, reserving 1 cup pasta water.

6. Stir the cream cheese and the marjoram into the bell pepper mixture. Purée using an immersion blender. You can also purée this sauce in batches in a blender or food processor. If you choose that method, return all the sauce to the skillet.

7. Add the cooked and drained pasta to the sauce along with enough reserved pasta water to make a smooth sauce that coats the pasta.

8. Sprinkle with the Parmesan cheese and serve.

Make It Easier Tip: You can substitute 1 (15-ounce) jar of roasted red bell peppers, drained, for the fresh peppers in this recipe.

Nutrition Info per Serving: Calories: 408; Total fat 19g; Saturated fat: 9g; Sodium: 188mg; Potassium: 330mg; Phosphorus: 222mg; Carbohydrates: 51g; Fiber: 6g; Protein: 12g; Sugar: 5g

Herbed Mushroom Burgers

DIABETES-FRIENDLY, LOW PROTEIN, HIGH FIBER

Serves 4 • Prep time: 20 minutes • Cook time: 10 minutes

Mushrooms have a taste and texture very similar to meat, so they are a great choice for vegetarian recipes. That's because they have a flavor called umami, *one of the five taste senses, that is savory and meaty. Lots of herbs accent these tasty burgers, which are served on whole-wheat buns with gravy made from pan drippings. Delicious!*

4 (4-ounce) cans no-salt-added mushroom pieces and stems, drained

3 scallions, white and green parts, cut into 1-inch pieces

2 garlic cloves, sliced

1 teaspoon dried Italian seasoning

1 large egg

⅔ cup crushed puffed rice cereal

2 tablespoons grated Parmesan cheese

2 tablespoons olive oil

1 tablespoon flour

1 cup low-sodium vegetable broth

4 whole-wheat hamburger buns, split and toasted

1. Combine the drained mushrooms, scallions, garlic, and Italian seasoning in a blender or food processor and blend or process until finely chopped.

2. Transfer the mushroom mixture to a medium bowl. Add the egg, crushed puffed rice cereal, and Parmesan cheese and mix.

3. Form the mixture into four ½-inch thick patties and set aside.

4. Heat the olive oil in a large skillet over medium heat.

5. Add the patties and cook, turning once carefully, for 3 to 4 minutes per side until hot, 160°F internal temperature.

6. Carefully remove the patties from the skillet to a plate and cover with foil to keep warm.

7. Add the flour to the drippings in the skillet and cook, stirring, for 1 minute. Stir in the broth and cook for 2 to 3 minutes longer or until the sauce thickens and bubbles.

8. Place the burgers on the buns and serve with the sauce poured over.

Increase Protein Tip: To make this a medium-protein recipe, add a slice of low-sodium Swiss cheese to each burger. The protein content will increase to 18 grams per serving.

Nutrition Info per Serving: Calories: 253; Total fat 11g; Saturated fat: 2g; Sodium: 305mg; Potassium: 315mg; Phosphorus: 218mg; Carbohydrates: 30g; Fiber: 6g; Protein: 11g; Sugar: 5g

Chickpea Curry

DIABETES-FRIENDLY, HIGH FIBER, LOW PROTEIN

Serves 4 • Prep time: 20 minutes • Cook time: 10 minutes

Chickpeas, also known as garbanzo beans, are nutty little nuggets with an impressive nutritional profile. They combine beautifully with tender cauliflower florets and pungent garlic in this satisfying meal served over rice. If you are new to the world of curry spices, reduce the curry powder to 1 teaspoon in this recipe. You can always add more!

2 tablespoons olive oil

1 onion, chopped

3 garlic cloves, minced

1 cup chopped
cauliflower florets

1 tablespoon
curry powder

1 (15-ounce) canned
no-salt-added or
low-sodium chickpeas,
rinsed and drained

1 cup low-sodium
vegetable broth

1 tablespoon freshly
squeezed lemon juice

Pinch salt

1 cup unsweetened
almond milk

2 tablespoons
cornstarch

2 cups cooked
brown rice

1. Heat the olive oil in a large skillet over medium heat.

2. Add the onion and garlic and sauté for 2 to 3 minutes or until tender-crisp.

3. Add the cauliflower, curry powder, and chickpeas; sauté for 1 minute.

4. Add the broth, lemon juice, and salt and bring to a simmer. Reduce the heat to low and simmer for 5 to 6 minutes or until the vegetables are tender.

5. In a small bowl, stir together the milk and cornstarch. Add this mixture to the skillet and cook, stirring constantly, for 2 minutes or until the sauce thickens and comes to a boil.

6. Serve the curry over the rice.

Increase Protein Tip: To make this a medium-protein recipe, add another ½ can drained chickpeas. The protein content will increase to 19 grams per serving.

Nutrition Info per Serving: Calories: 386; Total fat 12g; Saturated fat: 2g; Sodium: 137mg; Potassium: 425mg; Phosphorus: 232mg; Carbohydrates: 60g; Fiber: 10g; Protein: 12g; Sugar: 7g

Veggie Cabbage Stir-Fry

Serves 4 • Prep time: 20 minutes • Cook time: 10 minutes

Cabbage is a high-fiber, nutrient-dense vegetable, and an excellent ingredient for stir-fries. It cooks quickly and becomes tender and slightly sweet in the heat of the pan. This dish gets a wonderful color from the combination of vegetables, especially if you use both red and green cabbage.

1 cup low-sodium vegetable broth

1 tablespoon cornstarch

2 teaspoons low-sodium soy sauce

½ teaspoon ground ginger

2 tablespoons olive oil

4 cups chopped cabbage

1 (8-ounce) package sliced mushrooms

2 cups grated carrots

2 garlic cloves, sliced

3 cups cooked brown rice

1. In a small bowl, stir together the broth, cornstarch, soy sauce, and ginger; set aside.
2. Heat the olive oil in a wok or large skillet over medium heat.
3. Stir-fry the cabbage for 3 minutes.
4. Stir in the mushrooms, carrots, and garlic and stir-fry for another 2 minutes.
5. Add the broth mixture to the skillet. Stir until the sauce bubbles and thickens and the cabbage is tender, 4 to 5 minutes.
6. Serve the stir-fry over the rice.

Make It Easier Tip: To save time, you can use pre-shredded cabbage from the produce aisle in the supermarket. This product cooks more quickly, so only stir-fry for 1 minute in step 3.

Nutrition Info per Serving: Calories: 307; Total fat 9g; Saturated fat: 1g; Sodium: 174mg; Potassium: 579mg; Phosphorus: 247mg; Carbohydrates: 52g; Fiber: 6g; Protein: 8g; Sugar: 6g

Veggie Risotto

LOW PROTEIN, ONE POT

Serves 4 • Prep time: 5 minutes • Cook time: 25 minutes

Risotto is an elegant dish that is typically made with arborio rice, short-grain rice that comes from Italy. This rice becomes very creamy and rich when cooked because it releases loads of starch as it absorbs the broth and simmers. To make this recipe in 30 minutes, use pre-grated carrots and sliced mushrooms to reduce preparation time.

4 cups low-sodium
   vegetable broth
1 tablespoon olive oil
2 tablespoons unsalted
   butter, divided
1 (8-ounce) package
   sliced cremini
   mushrooms

1 cup grated carrots
3 garlic cloves, sliced
1 teaspoon dried
   Italian seasoning
1½ cups arborio rice or
   long-grain white rice

1 cup frozen baby peas
2 tablespoons grated
   Parmesan cheese

1. Pour the broth into a medium saucepan and bring to a simmer over high heat. Reduce the heat to low to keep it warm.

2. Meanwhile, heat the olive oil and 1 tablespoon butter in a large skillet over medium heat.

3. Add the mushrooms, carrots, and garlic. Sauté for 2 minutes, stirring frequently.

4. Stir in the Italian seasoning and the rice and sauté for 2 minutes longer.

5. Add the warm broth to the rice mixture, about ½ cup at a time, stirring constantly.

6. Each time the broth is absorbed, add more to the skillet. You can stir less often as the rice begins to cook, but keep an eye on the skillet.

7. When the broth is almost finished, stir the peas into the rice. The risotto is done when the rice is tender and most of the broth is absorbed. This whole process should take about 20 minutes. You may not need all of the broth. This dish can be soupier or thicker, depending on how much broth you add and your taste.

8. Stir in the remaining butter and the cheese and serve immediately.

Ingredient Tip: Long-grain white rice will work as a substitute in this recipe if you can't find arborio rice. Just keep stirring to help the rice release starch as it cooks.

Nutrition Info per Serving: Calories: 412; Total fat 11g; Saturated fat: 5g; Sodium: 255mg; Potassium: 535mg; Phosphorus: 217mg; Carbohydrates: 68g; Fiber: 4g; Protein: 10g; Sugar: 5g

Creamy Mac and Cheese

LOW PROTEIN, ONE POT

Serves 6 • Prep time: 15 minutes • Cook time: 15 minutes

While few can resist the comforting taste of creamy mac and cheese, people with CKD need to be cautious of the large amounts of sodium and phosphorus in the traditional recipe. The ingredients in this version have been adjusted to make it more suitable for the renal diet. It's still just as irresistible!

3 cups dry elbow
macaroni

3 cups low-sodium
vegetable broth

1 cup unsweetened
almond milk

½ cup shredded sharp
cheddar cheese

1 tablespoon cornstarch

1 (8-ounce) package
cream cheese, cubed

2 tablespoons grated
Parmesan cheese

1. Put the pasta, broth, and milk in a large saucepan over medium heat. Bring the liquid to a simmer and reduce the heat to low.
2. Cook, stirring frequently, for 8 to 9 minutes or until the pasta is almost al dente.
3. While the pasta is cooking, toss the cheddar cheese with the cornstarch in a small bowl.
4. When the pasta is cooked, stir the cream cheese, cheddar cheese mixture, and Parmesan into the pot.
5. Cook, stirring constantly, until the cheeses have melted and the sauce is creamy. Serve.

Increase Protein Tip: To make this a medium-protein recipe, add 1 scoop (2 tablespoons) of unflavored protein powder in step 1. Adding a protein powder with 30 grams protein per scoop will increase the protein content to 19 grams per serving.

Diabetes Tip: To make this a diabetes-friendly recipe, switch to whole-wheat elbow macaroni. The carbohydrate content will stay the same, but the fiber content will increase to 6 grams per serving.

Nutrition Info per Serving: Calories: 422; Total fat 18g; Saturated fat: 10g; Sodium: 317mg; Potassium: 245mg; Phosphorus: 219mg; Carbohydrates: 51g; Fiber: 2g; Protein: 14g; Sugar: 4g

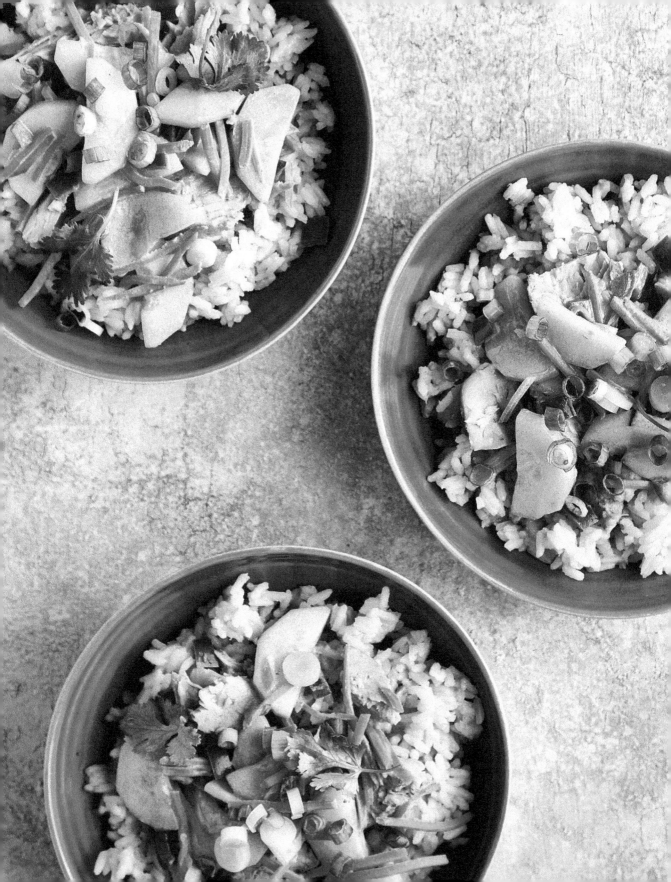

Seafood Entrées

⇦*Asian-Style Salmon and Rice Bowls, page 100*

Curried Fish Cakes

DIABETES-FRIENDLY, MEDIUM PROTEIN

Serves 4 • Prep time: 10 minutes • Cook time: 18 minutes

Thai curry paste and curry powder add a complex spiciness to this recipe, while the apple lends a touch of sweetness. Puffed rice cereal may seem like an unusual ingredient for fish cakes, but using cereal instead of breadcrumbs lowers the potassium and phosphorus content. Fish cakes are delicious served with steamed or sautéed vegetables.

¾ pound Atlantic cod, cubed

1 apple, peeled and cubed

1 tablespoon yellow curry paste

2 tablespoons cornstarch

1 tablespoon peeled grated ginger root

1 large egg

1 tablespoon freshly squeezed lemon juice

⅛ teaspoon freshly ground black pepper

½ cup crushed puffed rice cereal

1 tablespoon olive oil

1. Put the cod, apple, curry, cornstarch, ginger, egg, lemon juice, and pepper in a blender or food processor and process until finely chopped. Avoid over-processing, or the mixture will become mushy.

2. Place the rice cereal on a shallow plate.

3. Form the mixture into 8 patties.

4. Dredge the patties in the rice cereal to coat.

5. Heat the oil in a large skillet over medium heat.

6. Cook patties for 4 to 5 minutes per side, turning once until a meat thermometer registers 160°F.

7. Serve.

Increase Protein Tip: To make this a high-protein recipe, use a full pound of cod fillets. The protein content will increase to 28 grams per serving.

Nutrition Info per Serving: Calories: 188; Total fat: 6g; Saturated fat: 1g; Sodium: 150mg; Potassium: 292mg; Phosphorus: 150mg; Carbohydrates: 12g; Fiber: 1g; Protein: 21g; Sugar: 5g

Shrimp Fettuccine

DIABETES-FRIENDLY, HIGH FIBER, MEDIUM PROTEIN

Serves 6 • Prep time: 20 minutes • Cook time: 10 minutes

Shrimp's high cholesterol might concern you. However, research shows that dietary cholesterol is not harmful and does not increase the level of bad cholesterol in the blood. The most recent dietary guidelines no longer recommend that people limit their cholesterol intake to a specific amount. So, go ahead and enjoy this shrimp dish without worrying that it will have negative consequences on your heart.

2 tablespoons olive oil

1 leek, white and green parts, chopped

12 ounces whole-wheat fettuccine pasta

1 cup green beans, cut into 1-inch pieces

1 red bell pepper, chopped

½ pound medium raw shrimp, peeled and deveined

1 cup low-sodium vegetable broth

½ teaspoon dried thyme leaves

2 tablespoons chopped fresh chives

3 tablespoons grated Parmesan cheese

1. Bring a large pot of water to a boil.

2. Meanwhile, heat the olive oil in a large skillet over medium heat.

3. Sauté the leek for 2 minutes.

4. Add the pasta to the boiling water; cook according to package instructions, until the fettuccine is al dente.

5. Add the green beans and red bell pepper to the skillet and sauté for 2 minutes.

6. Add the shrimp to the skillet and sauté for 1 minute.

7. Drain the pasta, reserving ½ cup cooking water.

8. Add the pasta, broth, and thyme to the skillet and cook for 3 to 4 minutes or until the sauce reduces slightly and the shrimp curls and turns pink.

9. Sprinkle with the chives and cheese and serve.

Increase Protein Tip: To make this a high-protein recipe, use a full pound of shrimp. The protein content will increase to 28 grams per serving.

Nutrition Info per Serving: Calories: 310; Total fat: 6g; Saturated fat: 1g; Sodium: 130mg; Potassium: 340mg; Phosphorus: 274mg; Carbohydrates: 48g; Fiber: 6g; Protein: 19g; Sugar: 2g

Baked Sole with Caramelized Onion

DIABETES-FRIENDLY, MEDIUM PROTEIN

Serves 4 • Prep time: 10 minutes • Cook time: 20 minutes

Caramelized onions usually take at least an hour to prepare, with lots of stirring and supervision. By using the tricks in this recipe (no oil in the pan and baking soda), you can make them in about 15 minutes. The caramelized onions pair deliciously with the tender sole and colorful vegetables in this tempting recipe.

1 cup finely
    chopped onion
½ cup low-sodium
    vegetable broth
1 yellow summer
    squash, sliced

2 cups frozen
    broccoli florets
4 (3-ounce) fillets of sole
Pinch salt
2 tablespoons olive oil
Pinch baking soda

2 teaspoons avocado oil
1 teaspoon dried
    basil leaves

1. Preheat the oven to 425°F.

2. In a medium skillet over medium-high heat, add the onions. Cook for 1 minute; then, stirring constantly, cook for another 4 minutes.

3. Remove the onions from the heat.

4. Pour the broth into a baking sheet with a lip and arrange the squash and broccoli on the sheet in a single layer. Top the vegetables with the fish. Sprinkle the fish with the salt and drizzle everything with the olive oil.

5. Bake the fish and the vegetables for 10 minutes.

6. While the fish is baking, return the skillet with the onions to medium-high heat and stir in a pinch of baking soda. Stir in the avocado oil and cook for 5 minutes, stirring frequently, until the onions are dark brown.

7. Transfer the onions to a plate.

8. Remove the baking sheet from the oven and top the fish evenly with the onions. Sprinkle with the basil.

9. Return the fish to the oven and bake 8 to 10 minutes longer or until the fish flakes when tested with a fork and the vegetables are tender. Serve the fish on the vegetables.

Ingredient Tip: Frozen fillets can be very high in sodium because they are often frozen in brine. Avoid any frozen fish that provides more than 200 milligrams of sodium per serving. If in doubt, purchase fresh fish.

Nutrition Info per Serving: Calories: 200; Total fat: 11g; Saturated fat: 2g; Sodium: 320mg; Potassium: 537; Phosphorus: 331mg; Carbohydrates: 10g; Fiber: 3g; Protein: 16g; Sugar: 4g

Veggie Seafood Stir-Fry

DIABETES-FRIENDLY, MEDIUM PROTEIN

Serves 6 • Prep time: 12 minutes • Cook time: 18 minutes

This easy and quick stir-fry is full of color and flavor. The shrimp is an indulgent and delicious addition to this basic recipe, but you can also make it with one pound of cubed raw chicken breast. Just be sure to cook the chicken to 165°F for food safety reasons.

1 cup low-sodium vegetable or chicken broth

1 tablespoon cornstarch

½ teaspoon ground ginger

⅛ teaspoon red pepper flakes

2 tablespoons olive oil

1 onion, chopped

2 carrots, peeled and thinly sliced

1 pound medium raw shrimp, peeled and deveined

1 cup snow peas

2 tablespoons sesame oil

2 cups cooked brown rice

1. In a small bowl, combine the broth, cornstarch, ginger, and red pepper flakes and set aside.

2. Heat the oil in a wok or large skillet over medium-high heat.

3. Stir-fry the onion and carrots for 3 to 4 minutes until tender-crisp.

4. Add the shrimp and snow peas and stir-fry for 3 minutes longer or until the shrimp curl and turn pink.

5. Add the sauce and stir-fry for 1 to 2 minutes longer or until the sauce bubbles and thickens.

6. Drizzle with the sesame oil and serve over the rice.

Increase Protein Tip: To make this a high-protein recipe, add 2 cups of frozen, shelled edamame in step 4. The protein content will increase to 25 grams per serving.

Nutrition Info per Serving: Calories: 306; Total fat: 15g; Saturated fat: 2g; Sodium: 127mg; Potassium: 385mg; Phosphorus: 269mg; Carbohydrates: 24g; Fiber: 2g; Protein: 21g; Sugar: 3g

Thai Tuna Wraps

DIABETES-FRIENDLY, MEDIUM PROTEIN, ONE POT

Serves 4 • Prep time: 10 minutes

Wraps don't have to be made with tortillas or bread wrappers; lettuce leaves are a light and healthy alternative. Butter lettuce is very tender and mild, so it works well with the spicy filling. This fragrant veggie-and-tuna-packed wrap can be made with canned or cooked salmon, too.

¼ cup unsalted
   peanut butter
2 tablespoons freshly
   squeezed lemon juice
1 teaspoon low-sodium
   soy sauce
½ teaspoon
   ground ginger

⅛ teaspoon
   cayenne pepper
1 (6-ounce) can
   no-salt-added or
   low-sodium chunk
   light tuna, drained
1 cup shredded
   red cabbage

2 scallions, white and
   green parts, chopped
1 cup grated carrots
8 butter lettuce leaves

1. In a medium bowl, stir together the peanut butter, lemon juice, soy sauce, ginger, and cayenne pepper until well combined.

2. Stir in the tuna, cabbage, scallions, and carrots.

3. Divide the tuna filling evenly between the butter lettuce leaves and serve.

Ingredient Tip: Make sure to choose light tuna for this recipe, as other types of tuna can contain high amounts of mercury, a dangerous heavy metal. When possible, look for Safe Catch brand tuna because this company only uses fish that is 70 to 90 percent lower than the FDA's mercury limit for albacore tuna.

Reduce Protein Tip: To make this a low-protein recipe, decrease the tuna to 3 ounces and add 1 cup canned, drained low-sodium chickpeas. The protein content will drop to 13 grams per serving, and the recipe will become high fiber.

Nutrition Info per Serving: Calories: 172; Total fat; 9g; Saturated fat: 1g; Sodium: 98mg; Potassium: 421mg; Phosphorus: 153mg; Carbohydrates: 8g; Fiber: 2g; Protein: 17g; Sugar: 4g

Grilled Fish and Vegetable Packets

DIABETES-FRIENDLY, HIGH PROTEIN

Serves 4 • Prep time: 15 minutes • Cook time: 12 minutes

Did you know that you can grill fish fillets if you wrap them in foil? The delicate flesh can stick and tear if placed directly on the grill. These one-dish foil packets are great for entertaining or a quick weeknight dinner. Just place each packet on a plate and let your guests unwrap them; but be careful of the steam.

1 (8-ounce) package sliced mushrooms

1 leek, white and green parts, chopped

1 cup frozen corn

4 (4-ounce) Atlantic cod fillets

Juice of 1 lemon

3 tablespoons olive oil

1. Prepare and preheat the grill to medium coals and set a grill 6 inches from the coals.
2. Tear off four 30-inch long strips of heavy-duty aluminum foil.
3. Arrange the mushrooms, leek, and corn in the center of each piece of foil and top with the fish.
4. Drizzle the packet contents evenly with the lemon juice and olive oil.
5. Bring the longer length sides of the foil together at the top and, holding the edges together, fold them over twice and then fold in the width sides to form a sealed packet with room for the steam.
6. Put the packets on the grill and grill for 10 to 12 minutes until the vegetables are tender-crisp and the fish flakes when tested with a fork. Be careful opening the packets because the escaping steam can be scalding.

Make It Easier Tip: If you don't have a grill or you don't want to grill, you can bake these packets in the oven using parchment paper or foil. Put the packets on a baking sheet and bake at 450°F for 12 to 15 minutes.

Nutrition Info per Serving: Calories: 267; Total fat: 12g; Saturated fat: 2g; Sodium: 97mg; Potassium: 582mg; Phosphorus: 238mg; Carbohydrates: 13g; Fiber: 2g; Protein: 29g; Sugar: 3g

Scrambled Eggs with Crab

DIABETES-FRIENDLY, MEDIUM PROTEIN

Serves 4 • Prep time: 10 minutes • Cook time: 8 minutes

Scrambled eggs are not just for breakfast; they are delicious for dinner, too. Add some whole-wheat toast and fresh fruit for a pretty and filling meal. This sophisticated twist on the classic recipe is ready in minutes, so it is perfect for a quick dinner.

6 large eggs

4 egg whites

⅛ teaspoon freshly ground black pepper

2 tablespoons unsalted butter

1 red bell pepper, chopped

3 scallions, white and green parts, chopped

1 (6-ounce) can crab meat, drained

¼ cup shredded Swiss cheese

1 tablespoon chopped fresh chives

1. In a medium bowl, whisk together the eggs, egg whites, and pepper until well blended and set aside.

2. Melt the butter in a large skillet over medium heat.

3. Sauté the red bell pepper and scallions for 2 minutes. Stir in the crab and cook for 1 minute longer. Remove this mixture from the skillet to a plate and set aside.

4. Add the beaten eggs to the skillet and cook, stirring occasionally, until the eggs form large curds and are set, about 2 to 4 minutes.

5. Add the vegetables and crab back to the eggs. Sprinkle with the cheese and cover the skillet for 1 minute to melt the cheese.

6. Remove the cover, sprinkle with the chives, and serve.

Ingredient Tip: Canned seafood, including crab, often contains phosphate additives, so scan the ingredient list before purchasing. The Trader Joe's and Crown Prince brands of canned crab are both free of phosphate additives. These products tend to contain upward of 300mg of sodium per serving, so this recipe contains no added salt.

Increase Protein Tip: To make this a high-protein recipe, use six egg whites. The protein content will increase to 25 grams per serving.

Nutrition Info per Serving: Calories: 258; Total fat: 16g; Saturated fat: 7g; Sodium: 404mg; Potassium: 346mg; Phosphorus: 285mg; Carbohydrates: 4g; Fiber: 1g; Protein: 23g; Sugar: 3g

Baked Ginger Infused Cod

DIABETES-FRIENDLY, HIGH PROTEIN, ONE POT

Serves 4 • Prep time: 15 minutes • Cook time: 10 minutes

Ginger is a wonderful and fragrant ingredient to use with fish, and thanks to its low phosphorus content, cod fillets are a good seafood choice for people with CKD. This tender fish is delicious when brushed with olive oil, sprinkled with herbs, and baked in the oven with some summer squash.

4 (4-ounce) Atlantic cod fillets

2 tablespoons peeled and grated fresh ginger root

2 tablespoons olive oil, divided

1 lemon

1 yellow summer squash, sliced

Pinch salt

⅛ teaspoon freshly ground black pepper

½ teaspoon dried thyme leaves

1. Preheat the oven to 400°F. Pat the fillets dry with a paper towel and sprinkle them with the ginger root.

2. Spread 1 tablespoon of the olive oil in a 12-by-8-inch baking dish.

3. Thinly slice half of the lemon, remove the seeds from the slices, and arrange the slices in the baking dish in a single layer.

4. Top the lemon slices with the squash slices.

5. Place the fish on top of the squash and sprinkle with the salt, pepper, and thyme. Drizzle with the remaining olive oil and squeeze the juice from the remaining lemon half on the fish.

6. Bake the cod for 12 to 15 minutes, or until the fish registers at least 145°F on a meat thermometer and flakes when tested with a fork. Serve with the squash and lemon slices.

Ingredient Tip: To grate ginger root, first peel the knobby root with a vegetable peeler or the side of a spoon. Grate the ginger on the fine side of a box grater.

Reduce Protein Tip: To make this a medium-protein recipe, use 3-ounce fish fillets. The protein content will decrease to 20 grams per serving.

Nutrition Info per Serving: Calories: 194; Total fat: 8g; Saturated fat: 1g; Sodium: 132mg; Potassium: 449mg; Phosphorus: 179mg; Carbohydrates: 4g; Fiber: 1g; Protein: 27g; Sugar: 2g

Spicy Wild Salmon Wraps

DIABETES-FRIENDLY, MEDIUM PROTEIN, ONE POT

Serves 4 • Prep time: 15 minutes

Salmon is a low-mercury fish high in anti-inflammatory omega-3 fatty acids. Farmed salmon, as opposed to wild, is high in contaminants, and these may pose risks to your health. While it's true that wild salmon contains more potassium than farmed salmon, this recipe keeps potassium levels down by using only 2 ounces of wild salmon per serving. That portion size contains more than the daily-recommended amount of omega-3 fatty acids. It's a win-win!

4 ounces cream cheese, softened

2 tablespoons freshly squeezed lemon juice

8 ounces canned wild salmon, drained

1 jalapeño pepper, minced

2 cups shredded coleslaw mix

4 (6-inch) corn tortillas

1. In a medium bowl, beat the cream cheese and lemon juice with a spoon until smooth.
2. Stir in the salmon, jalapeño pepper, and coleslaw mix until well combined
3. Evenly divide the salmon filling between the corn tortillas, wrap them up, and serve.

Ingredient Tip: Corn tortillas need to be softened before you can roll them. To soften, wrap them in damp microwave-safe paper towels and microwave on high power for 1 minute or until the tortillas are soft.

Reduce Protein Tip: To make this a low-protein recipe, reduce the salmon to 6 ounces and add ½ cup shredded lettuce to each wrap to create bulk. The protein content will decrease to 14 grams per serving.

Nutrition Info per Wrap: Calories: 267; Total fat: 15g; Saturated fat: 7g; Sodium: 138mg; Potassium: 519mg; Phosphorus: 262mg; Carbohydrates: 15g; Fiber: 2g; Protein: 18g; Sugar: 3g

Tuna Fruit Salad

Serves 4 • Prep time: 10 minutes

Canned chunk light tuna is a convenient and inexpensive option for seafood recipes. The fish is combined with fresh apples and blueberries in this colorful and nutritious take on traditional tuna salad. Try serving it with whole-grain crackers, or over a bed of lettuce. You can also make this recipe with canned salmon or even crab for a decadent variation.

½ cup part skim ricotta cheese

Juice of 1 lemon

½ teaspoon dried marjoram leaves

1 (5-ounce) can no-salt-added or low-sodium chunk light tuna, drained

1 Granny Smith apple, chopped

1 cup blueberries

2 celery stalks, chopped

1. In a medium bowl, stir together the ricotta, lemon juice, and marjoram leaves.

2. Stir in the tuna, apple, blueberries, and celery until well mixed.

3. Serve.

Increase Protein Tip: To make this a medium-protein recipe, add 1 cup of thawed, frozen shelled edamame beans. The protein content will increase to 18 grams per serving.

Nutrition Info per Serving: Calories: 135; Total fat: 3g; Saturated fat: 2g; Sodium: 65mg; Potassium: 265mg; Phosphorus: 129mg; Carbohydrates:14g; Fiber: 2g; Protein: 13g; Sugar: 8g

Sole Scampi Bake

DIABETES-FRIENDLY, MEDIUM PROTEIN

Serves 4 • Prep time: 14 minutes • Cook time: 16 minutes

While scampi is technically large shrimp or prawns, it can also describe seafood that is cooked in lemon butter and garlic sauce. Typically an uncomplicated recipe, this variation is dressed up with lots of fresh, colorful, and delicious vegetables, so the presentation is spectacular, and the dish is especially nutrient-dense.

1 lemon

3 tablespoons unsalted butter

3 garlic cloves, thinly sliced

1 red bell pepper, sliced

16 asparagus spears, trimmed

3 celery stalks, sliced

4 (3-ounce) sole fillets

Pinch salt

⅛ teaspoon freshly ground black pepper

1. Preheat the oven to 400°F.

2. Zest 1 teaspoon lemon zest and squeeze the lemon, reserving the juice in a small bowl.

3. Melt the butter in a small skillet over medium heat and sauté the garlic until fragrant, 1 minute.

4. Remove the skillet from the heat and stir in the lemon zest and reserved lemon juice.

5. Place the bell pepper, asparagus, and celery on a baking sheet with a lip. Top the vegetables with the fish and sprinkle with the salt and pepper.

6. Pour the garlic mixture over the fish and vegetables.

7. Bake for 12 to 16 minutes or until the vegetables are tender-crisp and the fish flakes when tested with a fork.

8. Serve the vegetables and fish together.

Ingredient Tip: To prepare fresh asparagus, bend each spear until it snaps. The spear will break naturally at the point where it becomes tough.

Nutrition Info per Serving: Calories: 186; Total fat: 9g; Saturated fat: 6g; Sodium: 289mg; Potassium: 431mg; Phosphorus: 270mg; Carbohydrates: 7g; Fiber: 3g; Protein: 13g; Sugar: 3g

Mackerel Mushroom Risotto

LOW PROTEIN, ONE POT

Serves 6 • Prep time: 8 minutes • Cook time: 22 minutes

Salmon and tuna might be more familiar, but mackerel is a rich and flavorful fish that's very high in anti-inflammatory omega-3 fatty acids. Look for canned Atlantic mackerel instead of King, Spanish, or Gulf mackerel because these other products contain high amounts of mercury.

4 cups low-sodium
   vegetable broth
1 (4.4-ounce) can
   Atlantic mackerel in oil
1 onion, chopped

1 (8-ounce)
   package sliced
   cremini mushrooms
2 garlic cloves, minced
1½ cups arborio rice or
   long-grain white rice

Juice of 1 lemon
2 tablespoons
   unsalted butter
2 tablespoon grated
   Parmesan cheese

1. Bring the broth to a simmer in a small saucepan over low heat. Set aside and cover to keep warm.

2. Drain the mackerel, reserving the oil. Put 2 tablespoons of the oil into a large saucepan and heat over medium heat.

3. Add the onion and mushrooms and sauté for 2 minutes.

4. Stir in the garlic and rice and sauté for 2 minutes.

5. Start adding the broth to the rice mixture, about ½ cup at a time, stirring constantly.

6. When the broth is absorbed, add more broth. You can stir less often as the rice begins to cook but keep an eye on the pan.

7. The risotto is done when the rice is tender and most of the broth is absorbed, about 20 minutes in total. You may not need all of the broth. This dish can be soupier or thicker, depending on how much broth you add and your taste.

8. Stir in the reserved mackerel, lemon juice, butter, and cheese and serve immediately.

Ingredient Tip: You can purchase good-quality canned mackerel, in addition to other fish, online. Wild Planet Foods (WildPlanetFoods.com) or Vital Choice (Vital-Choice.com) are both good brands.

Nutrition Info per Serving: Calories: 270; Total fat: 6g; Saturated fat: 3g; Sodium: 213mg; Potassium: 334mg; Phosphorus: 187mg; Carbohydrates: 43g; Fiber: 1g; Protein: 10g; Sugar: 2g

Creamy Clam and Mushroom Pasta

MEDIUM PROTEIN

Serves 6 • Prep time: 15 minutes • Cook time: 15 minutes

This is not a traditional cream-heavy pasta and clams recipe. It is lighter and filled with loads of colorful, nutritious vegetables. The dish is still elegant enough for company but is also the perfect choice for a busy weeknight when you want to treat yourself. Clams are an excellent source of iron, which is important because many people with CKD are iron deficient.

8 ounces small
  shell pasta
2 tablespoons olive oil
1 onion, chopped
1 (8-ounce) package
  sliced button
  mushrooms
1 red bell pepper,
  chopped

1½ cups baby
  frozen peas
½ teaspoon dried
  basil leaves
1 cup low-sodium
  vegetable broth
1 (6-ounce) can
  clams, drained

½ cup part skim
  ricotta cheese
½ cup shredded
  mozzarella cheese

1. Bring a large pot of water to a boil. Add the pasta; cook according to package directions until the pasta is just al dente. Drain, reserving ½ cup pasta cooking water.

2. While the pasta is cooking, heat the olive oil in a large skillet over medium heat.

3. Add the onion and mushrooms and sauté for 3 minutes.

4. Stir in the bell pepper, peas, and basil and sauté 1 minute longer.

5. Add the vegetable broth and clams and bring to a simmer.

6. Simmer the sauce for 3 minutes and stir in the ricotta cheese until the sauce is creamy.

7. Add the pasta and mozzarella cheese and stir until creamy, adding reserved pasta cooking water if necessary.

8. Serve.

Ingredient Tip: Canned clams do contain added salt, so no extra salt is needed in this recipe. When shopping, look for Crown Prince or Trader Joe's brand of canned clams since they are free of phosphate additives.

Nutrition Info per Serving: Calories: 309; Total fat: 9g; Saturated fat: 3g; Sodium: 307mg; Potassium: 449mg; Phosphorus: 299mg; Carbohydrates: 39g; Fiber: 4g; Protein: 18g; Sugar: 5g

Asian-Style Salmon and Rice Bowls

MEDIUM PROTEIN

Serves 4 • Prep time: 10 minutes • Cook time: 20 minutes

Dinner bowls are tasty creations that usually contain a combination of rice or beans, protein, and vegetables. This recipe combines Asian flavors such as lime and ginger, salmon, and rice with sautéed cucumber. If you have never cooked cucumber, you are in for a treat because it becomes tender and slightly sweet.

1½ cups long grain white rice

3 cups low-sodium vegetable broth

2 tablespoons olive oil

1 cup grated carrots

1 cucumber, peeled and sliced

1 jalapeño pepper, minced

2 teaspoons low-sodium soy sauce

2 tablespoons mayonnaise

1 tablespoon freshly squeezed lime juice

½ teaspoon ground ginger

1 (5-ounce) can wild salmon, drained

1. In a medium saucepan, combine the rice and broth and bring to a boil over high heat. Reduce the heat to low and simmer for 18 to 20 minutes or until the rice is tender and the liquid is absorbed.

2. While the rice is cooking, heat the olive oil in a small saucepan over medium heat.

3. Sauté the carrot, cucumber, and jalapeño pepper for 3 to 4 minutes or until the vegetables are tender.

4. Stir in the soy sauce, mayonnaise, lime juice, and ground ginger and heat for 1 minute.

5. Divide the rice among four bowls and top with the salmon and then the vegetable mixture. Serve.

Ingredient Tip: You can make the rice for this bowl ahead of time. Refrigerate it promptly after cooking and reheat thoroughly in the microwave; or you can use frozen rice prepared according to package directions.

Nutrition Info per Bowl: Calories: 431; Total fat: 13g; Saturated fat: 2g; Sodium: 287mg; Potassium: 522mg; Phosphorus: 203mg; Carbohydrates: 62g; Fiber: 2g; Protein: 15g; Sugar: 3g

Persian Fish

DIABETES-FRIENDLY, HIGH PROTEIN

Serves 4 • Prep time: 10 minutes • Cook time: 15 minutes

Persian ingredients are easy to find in most grocery stores, and those products are combined in a unique and delicious fish dish here. This recipe puts together macadamia nuts, grapes, lime juice, onion, cinnamon, and turmeric for a flavorful, fragrant, colorful meal that is quick to prepare and pleasing to eat.

½ teaspoon ground turmeric

½ teaspoon ground cinnamon

¼ teaspoon onion powder

2 tablespoons freshly squeezed lime juice

2 tablespoons olive oil

2 cups seedless red grapes

3 celery stalks, sliced

4 (4-ounce) Atlantic cod fillets

½ cup ground macadamia nuts

1. Preheat the oven to 400°F.
2. In a small bowl, combine the turmeric, cinnamon, onion powder, and lime juice and set aside.
3. Grease a baking sheet with a lip with the olive oil and arrange the grapes and celery in a single layer and top with the fish fillets.
4. Brush the fish with the lime juice mixture and sprinkle with the macadamia nuts, pressing the nuts gently into the fish.
5. Bake for 15 to 18 minutes or until the fish flakes when tested with a fork.
6. Serve the fish with the grapes and celery.

Make It Easier Tip: Use 1½ teaspoons of your favorite curry powder instead of the turmeric, cinnamon, and onion powder in this recipe.

Nutrition Info per Serving: Calories: 293; Total fat: 13g; Saturated fat: 2g; Sodium: 129mg; Potassium: 595mg; Phosphorus: 199mg; Carbohydrates: 18g; Fiber: 2g; Protein: 27g; Sugar: 13g

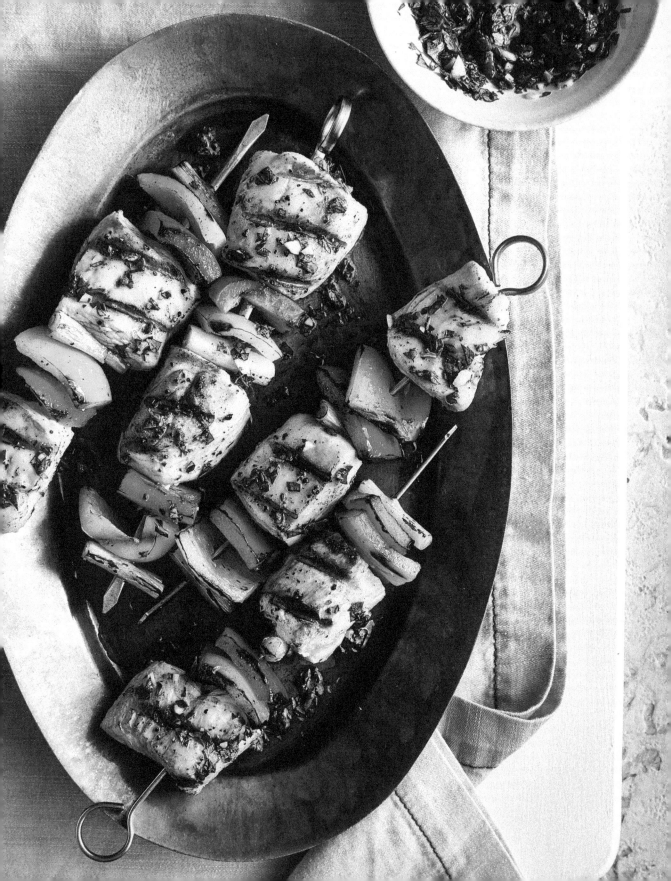

Poultry and Meat Entrées

⇦*Grilled Chimichurri Chicken Kebabs, page 110*

Barley Chicken Salad

Serves 6 • Prep time: 20 minutes • Cook time: 6 minutes

Barley is a grain with a mild, slightly nutty flavor and pleasantly chewy texture. It is combined with tender chicken breast, a simple vinaigrette, and heaps of vegetables in this satisfying and delicious one-dish meal. The dressing is one that can be made separately in a larger quantity and used on other salads.

¾ cup quick-cooking barley

2½ cups low-sodium chicken broth

5 tablespoons olive oil, divided

12 ounces boneless skinless chicken breasts, cubed

Juice of 1 lemon

1 tablespoon yellow mustard

½ teaspoon dried oregano leaves

1 cucumber, peeled and sliced

1 red bell pepper, chopped

1 cup frozen corn, thawed and drained

1. In a medium saucepan over high heat, combine the barley and chicken broth and bring to a simmer.

2. Reduce the heat to low, partially cover the pan, and simmer for 10 to 12 minutes or until the barley is tender.

3. While the barley is cooking, heat 2 tablespoons olive oil in a medium skillet over medium heat.

4. Add the chicken and cook, stirring occasionally, until the chicken is fully cooked to 165°F internal temperature, 5 to 6 minutes. Remove the skillet from the heat.

5. In a serving bowl, whisk the remaining 3 tablespoons olive oil, lemon juice, mustard, and oregano until blended.

6. Add the cooked chicken, barley, cucumber, bell pepper, and corn and toss to coat.

7. This salad can be served warm or chilled in the refrigerator for 2 hours first.

Ingredient Tip: Use caution when working with raw chicken. This meat is often contaminated with pathogens such as salmonella, and people with chronic illnesses are more likely to suffer complications from an infection. Work on a cutting board separate from the one you use to prepare vegetables and always cook chicken to 165°F and use a food thermometer. Wash your hands thoroughly with soap and water after handling raw chicken.

Nutrition Info per Serving: Calories: 281; Total fat: 14g; Saturated fat: 2g; Sodium: 87mg; Potassium: 475mg; Phosphorus: 220mg; Carbohydrates: 22g; Fiber: 3g; Protein: 18g; Sugar: 2g

Chicken Coleslaw Salad

DIABETES-FRIENDLY, LOW PROTEIN

Serves 6 • Prep time: 20 minutes • Cook time: 10 minutes

While traditional American meals usually include vegetables, meat is often the larger portion on the plate. This recipe flips that dynamic and shows how the opposite ratio, more veggies than protein, can be fantastic and satisfying. In this dish, crunchy cabbage and carrots are accented by a small amount of chicken and a tasty creamy mustard dill dressing.

2 tablespoons olive oil

12 ounces boneless skinless chicken breasts, cubed

Pinch salt

⅛ teaspoon freshly ground black pepper

⅓ cup mayonnaise

2 tablespoons mustard

Juice of 1 lemon

1 teaspoon dried dill weed

3 cups chopped red cabbage

3 cups chopped green cabbage

1½ cups grated carrots

1. Heat a medium skillet over medium heat and add the olive oil.

2. Season the chicken with the salt and pepper and add to the skillet. Sauté the chicken until it is fully cooked to 165°F internal temperature. Remove the chicken from the skillet with a slotted spoon to a clean plate and set aside.

3. In a serving bowl, stir together the mayonnaise, mustard, lemon juice, and dill weed until well mixed.

4. Stir in the chicken, red cabbage, green cabbage, and carrots and toss to coat.

5. Serve immediately or cover and chill up to 2 hours before serving.

Make It Easier Tip: Instead of using raw chicken and cooking it from scratch, you can purchase a rotisserie chicken from the store and use the white meat to make this recipe. Because rotisserie chicken is prepared with salt, the sodium content of the recipe will increase to about 400 milligrams per serving.

Nutrition Info per Serving: Calories: 229; Total fat: 15g; Saturated fat: 2g; Sodium: 197mg; Potassium: 463mg; Phosphorus: 162mg; Carbohydrates: 9g; Fiber: 3g; Protein: 14g; Sugar: 4g

Berry-Chicken Pasta Salad

DIABETES-FRIENDLY, HIGH FIBER, MEDIUM PROTEIN

Serves 6 • Prep time: 20 minutes • Cook time: 6 minutes

Fruit might seem like an unusual addition to a savory pasta salad, but the sweetness and gorgeous color elevate this simple dish to something sublime. Whole-wheat pasta adds fiber and texture to this quick and tasty salad along with B-vitamins and iron, and the splash of lemon juice brightens up all the flavors.

8 ounces whole-wheat ziti or penne pasta

5 tablespoons olive oil, divided

12 ounces boneless skinless chicken breasts, cubed

Pinch salt

⅛ teaspoon freshly ground black pepper

Juice of 1 lemon

2 teaspoons honey

½ teaspoon dried thyme leaves

2 cups blueberries

1 cup sliced strawberries

1 cup raspberries

1. Bring a large pot of water to a boil. Add the pasta and cook according to package directions until al dente. Drain and set aside.

2. While the pasta is cooking, heat 2 tablespoons of olive oil in a medium skillet over medium heat.

3. Season the chicken with the salt and pepper and add to the skillet. Sauté for 5 to 6 minutes or until the chicken is thoroughly cooked to 165°F internal temperature. Remove the chicken from the skillet with a slotted spoon to a clean plate.

4. In a serving bowl, whisk the remaining 3 tablespoons of olive oil, lemon juice, honey, and thyme leaves until blended.

5. Stir in the cooked pasta, chicken, blueberries, and strawberries until combined.

6. Just before serving, top with the raspberries.

Ingredient Tip: All berries, and in fact all fresh produce, should be rinsed under cool running water before eating or slicing.

Nutrition Info per Serving: Calories: 357; Total fat: 14g; Saturated fat: 2g; Sodium: 55mg; Potassium: 472mg; Phosphorus: 269mg; Carbohydrates: 42g; Fiber: 7g; Protein: 19g; Sugar: 10g

Mexican-Style Chicken Salad

DIABETES-FRIENDLY, LOW PROTEIN

Serves 6 • Prep time: 20 minutes • Cook time: 8 minutes

Chicken is combined with lettuce, veggies, spices, and crunchy crushed tortilla chips for a flavor and texture explosion. The chili powder, cayenne pepper, and jalapeño add a triple dose of heat, so if you prefer a milder salad, you should reduce these ingredients to a comfortable level for your palate. The salad will still be delicious!

4 tablespoons olive oil, divided

12 ounces boneless skinless chicken thighs, cubed

3 teaspoons chili powder, divided

⅛ teaspoon cayenne pepper

2 tablespoons freshly squeezed lime juice

3 cups butter lettuce

1 red bell pepper, chopped

1½ cups frozen corn, thawed and drained

1 jalapeño pepper, minced

1 cup crushed yellow tortilla chips

½ cup Powerhouse Salsa (page 147)

1. Heat two tablespoons of oil in a medium skillet over medium heat.

2. Sprinkle the chicken thighs with 1 teaspoon chili powder and the cayenne pepper and cook, stirring frequently, for 6 to 8 minutes or until the chicken registers 165°F internal temperature.

3. Transfer the chicken to a serving bowl and add the remaining olive oil, remaining chili powder, and the lime juice. Toss to combine.

4. Add the butter lettuce, bell pepper, corn, and jalapeño pepper and toss.

5. Top with the tortilla chips and the salsa and serve

Ingredient Tip: Make sure you check the ingredient label and sodium content on the tortilla chips. Look for plain tortilla chips, not the high-sodium kind coated in a cheese or seasoning blend.

Nutrition Info per Serving: Calories: 270; Total fat: 15g; Saturated fat: 2g; Sodium: 161mg; Potassium: 489mg; Phosphorus: 186mg; Carbohydrates: 22g; Fiber: 4g; Protein: 14g; Sugar: 4g

Satay-Inspired Chicken Salad

DIABETES-FRIENDLY, MEDIUM PROTEIN

Serves 5 • Prep time: 20 minutes • Cook time: 6 minutes

Satay is an Indonesian dish that is usually made of chicken or pork, accompanied by a spicy peanut sauce. The chicken is grilled on skewers, but in this recipe, the chicken cooks in a skillet for ease of preparation. This recipe transforms the traditional version of satay into a main dish salad bursting with color and flavor.

3 tablespoons olive oil, divided

12 ounces boneless skinless chicken breasts, cubed

⅛ teaspoon cayenne pepper

⅓ cup crunchy peanut butter

¼ cup low-sodium chicken broth

Juice of 1 lemon

⅛ teaspoon red pepper flakes

1 cup grated carrot

3 scallions, white and green parts, sliced

2 cups chopped iceberg lettuce

2 cups chopped red cabbage

1. Heat 2 tablespoons of olive oil in a medium skillet over medium heat.
2. Sprinkle the chicken with cayenne pepper and add to the skillet.
3. Sauté the chicken until the chicken is cooked to 165°F internal temperature, between 5 and 8 minutes. Transfer the chicken to a clean plate and set aside.
4. In a medium bowl, whisk the peanut butter, broth, lemon juice, red pepper flakes, and the remaining olive oil until blended.
5. Stir in the chicken, carrot, and scallions until well mixed.
6. Place the lettuce and cabbage into a serving bowl and toss to combine. Top with the chicken mixture, toss it all together, and serve.

Reduce Protein Tip: To make this a low-protein recipe, decrease the chicken to 6 ounces. The protein content will decrease to 13 grams per serving. Feel free to increase the amount of vegetables.

Nutrition Info per Serving: Calories: 284; Total fat: 19g; Saturated fat: 3g; Sodium: 135mg; Potassium: 544mg; Phosphorus: 231mg; Carbohydrates: 10g; Fiber: 3g; Protein: 20g; Sugar: 5g

Grilled Chimichurri Chicken Kebabs

DIABETES-FRIENDLY, MEDIUM PROTEIN

Serves 4 • Prep time: 20 minutes • Cook time: 10 minutes

Chicken kebabs grilled with vegetables and chimichurri sauce are an inspired entrée choice for summer entertaining. Cut the vegetables into 1-inch pieces, roughly the same size as the chicken, so they cook evenly. Chimichurri sauce is a fragrant recipe from Argentina that is made with fresh herbs, oil, garlic, and lemon juice.

12 ounces boneless skinless chicken breasts, cubed

Pinch salt

⅛ teaspoon freshly ground black pepper

1 red bell pepper, cubed

1 yellow bell pepper, cubed

3 scallions, white and green parts, cut into 1-inch pieces

½ cup chopped flat-leaf parsley

¼ cup chopped cilantro

2 garlic cloves, minced

3 tablespoons extra-virgin olive oil, divided

1 tablespoon red wine vinegar

1. Prepare and preheat the grill to medium coals and set a grill 6 inches from the coals.

2. Sprinkle the chicken breast cubes with salt and pepper.

3. Thread the chicken, red bell pepper, yellow bell pepper, and scallions onto 8-inch metal skewers, alternating pieces of chicken with the veggies. Refrigerate.

4. In a small bowl, stir together the parsley, cilantro, garlic, 2 tablespoons olive oil, and the vinegar until well mixed.

5. Brush the kebabs with the remaining 1 tablespoon olive oil and grill, turning once, until the chicken is cooked to 165°F internal temperature and the vegetables are tender, 7 to 9 minutes.

6. Place the kebabs on a serving plate and drizzle with the sauce.

7. Serve.

Cooking Tip: Make sure the grill rack is very clean before you add the kebabs. Clean the grill after each use while it's still warm for best results, so the food doesn't stick. To clean, you can rub the cooled grill with crumpled foil or follow the manufacturer's instructions.

Increase Protein Tip: To make this a high-protein recipe, increase the chicken to 18 ounces. The protein content will increase to 25 grams per serving.

Nutrition Info per Serving: Calories: 217; Total fat: 13g; Saturated fat: 2g; Sodium: 86mg; Potassium: 479mg; Phosphorus: 206mg; Carbohydrates: 5g; Fiber: 1g; Protein: 20g; Sugar: 3g

Roasted Herb and Lemon Chicken with Mashed Sweet Potatoes

DIABETES-FRIENDLY, HIGH FIBER, HIGH PROTEIN

Serves 4 • Prep time: 10 minutes • Cook time: 20 minutes

Roasted chicken doesn't have to be whole breasts or an entire bird. It can be tasty cubes of meat cooked quickly, accompanied by tender beans and topped with herbs and fresh lemon. Delicious and time-efficient. Sweet potatoes are considered a high-potassium root vegetable, but double-boiling this ingredient lowers the potassium content by about 50 percent.

4 medium sweet potatoes, peeled and quartered

4 (4-ounce) boneless skinless chicken thighs

1 onion, cut into ½-inch pieces

1½ cups frozen green beans

3 tablespoons olive oil

Juice of 1 lemon

1 teaspoon dried basil leaves

½ teaspoon dried thyme leaves

½ teaspoon salt, divided

¼ teaspoon freshly ground black pepper, divided

1 tablespoon unsalted butter

½ teaspoon cinnamon

1. Preheat the oven to 450°F.

2. Bring a large pot of water to a boil and boil the sweet potatoes for 10 minutes.

3. Drain the potatoes, add more fresh water to the pot, and boil again until soft, about 10 minutes more.

4. While the sweet potatoes are boiling, pat the chicken dry with paper towels; do not rinse. Cut the chicken into cubes.

5. Arrange the chicken, onion, and green beans on a baking sheet with a lip.

6. Drizzle with the olive oil and lemon juice and sprinkle with the basil, thyme, half the salt, and half the pepper. Toss to coat and rearrange in a single layer.

7. Roast for 15 to 20 minutes or until the chicken registers 165°F internal temperature and the vegetables are tender-crisp.

8. When the sweet potatoes are done, drain and mash them with the butter, cinnamon, and the remaining salt and pepper. Serve with the chicken and vegetables.

Ingredient Tip: Never rinse chicken or any raw meat before preparing. Rinsing does not remove bacteria. The only way to make raw meat safe is to cook it thoroughly. In fact, rinsing chickens can spread bacteria around your kitchen since the water stream can aerosolize the pathogens. Just pat the chicken dry with paper towels and start cooking.

Nutrition Info per Serving: Calories: 400; Total fat: 18g; Saturated fat: 5g; Sodium: 485mg; Potassium: 590mg; Phosphorus: 284mg; Carbohydrates: 34g; Fiber: 6g; Protein: 26g; Sugar: 11g

Chicken and Broccoli Pan Bake

DIABETES-FRIENDLY, HIGH PROTEIN, ONE POT

Serves 4 • Prep time: 5 minutes • Cook time: 25 minutes

Chicken and broccoli is a classic combination used in many cuisines around the world. In this American recipe, dinner is made in one pan, making cleanup quick and easy. This simple recipe uses just a few ingredients, but the resulting meal is nourishing and filling. And who doesn't like only five minutes of prep and the rest of the work for dinner done in the oven with no supervision?

16 ounces boneless skinless chicken breasts, cubed

1½ cups frozen broccoli florets

2 cups frozen sliced carrots

4 tablespoons olive oil

Juice of 1 lemon

1 teaspoon dried oregano leaves

1. Preheat the oven to 450°F.
2. Arrange the chicken, broccoli, and carrots on a baking sheet with a lip.
3. Drizzle with the olive oil and lemon juice and sprinkle with the oregano. Toss to coat and arrange everything in a single layer.
4. Roast for 15 to 20 minutes until the chicken registers 165°F internal temperature and the vegetables are tender-crisp.
5. Serve.

Ingredient Tip: Many other frozen vegetables can be used in this simple one-sheet recipe. Try green beans, radishes, yellow summer squash, or asparagus.

Nutrition Info per Serving: Calories: 282; Total fat: 17g; Saturated fat: 3g; Sodium: 85mg; Potassium: 578mg; Phosphorus: 276mg; Carbohydrates: 6g; Fiber: 2g; Protein: 27g; Sugar: 2g

Moroccan Chicken and Vegetable Stew

DIABETES-FRIENDLY, HIGH FIBER, HIGH PROTEIN, ONE POT

Serves 4 • Prep time: 17 minutes • Cook time: 13 minutes

Chicken tagine is a slow-cooked Moroccan dish that is prepared in a clay pot that keeps all the juices and flavor inside the vessel, creating a tender and moist meal. This recipe shows you how to prepare a quicker version of the traditional dish using a skillet with a lid. The chicken basically braises with lots of flavorful ingredients such as garlic, ginger, cumin, turmeric, and vegetables.

2 tablespoons olive oil

12 ounces boneless skinless chicken thighs, cubed

1 onion, chopped

4 garlic cloves, minced

2 cups baby carrots

1 cup low-sodium chicken broth

1 teaspoon ground ginger

1 teaspoon ground cumin

½ teaspoon paprika

½ teaspoon ground turmeric

Pinch salt

⅛ teaspoon freshly ground black pepper

1½ cups frozen baby peas

1. Heat the olive oil in a large skillet over medium heat.

2. Add the chicken and onion and sauté for 3 minutes or until the chicken begins to brown.

3. Stir in the garlic, carrots, and chicken broth and bring to a simmer.

4. Reduce the heat to low and stir in the ginger, cumin, paprika, turmeric, salt, and pepper. Partially cover and simmer for 6 minutes.

5. Add the peas and simmer for 2 to 4 minutes longer or until the chicken registers 165°F internal temperature and the vegetables are tender-crisp.

6. Serve.

Make It Easier Tip: If you regularly use a lot of garlic, you can speed preparation time by using a specialty garlic press. You just put the whole, unpeeled garlic clove in the device and press. The skin is removed, and the garlic is minced in seconds.

Nutrition Info per Serving: Calories: 295; Total fat: 11g; Saturated fat: 2g; Sodium: 239mg; Potassium: 584mg; Phosphorus: 267mg; Carbohydrates: 18g; Fiber: 5g; Protein: 30g; Sugar: 7g

Mushroom Turkey Burgers with Powerhouse Salsa

DIABETES-FRIENDLY, MEDIUM PROTEIN

Serves 4 • Prep time: 20 minutes • Cook time: 10 minutes

Finely chopped mushrooms add flavor and moisture to lean turkey, which tends to be dry when it's cooked to a safe temperature because it has so little fat. Serve these tender and delicious burgers on lettuce leaves and top with some flavorful home-made Powerhouse Salsa (page 147) for a satisfying dinner that's easy to make.

1 (8-ounce) package sliced cremini mushrooms

2 tablespoons olive oil

1 small onion, diced

½ pound 93-percent-lean ground turkey

1 large egg

3 tablespoons crushed puffed rice cereal

1 teaspoon dried thyme leaves

2 tablespoons unsalted butter

4 butter lettuce leaves

¼ cup Powerhouse Salsa (page 147)

1. Finely chop the mushrooms in a blender, food processor, or by hand.
2. Heat the olive oil in a large skillet over medium heat. Add the finely chopped mushrooms and onion and sauté, stirring frequently, until the mushrooms have given up their liquid, about 5 to 6 minutes.
3. Remove the mushrooms from the skillet and place in a medium bowl.
4. In another bowl, mix together the ground turkey, egg, crushed puffed rice cereal, and thyme leaves.
5. Mix in the mushroom mixture until well combined and form into 4 patties.
6. Heat the butter in a large skillet over medium heat.
7. Add the turkey patties and cook until they reach 165°F internal temperature, turning once, about 4 minutes per side.
8. Put each patty on a lettuce leaf and top each with 1 tablespoon of the salsa. Serve.

Nutrition Info per Burger with Salsa: Calories: 285; Total fat: 21g; Saturated fat: 7g; Sodium: 83mg; Potassium: 568mg; Phosphorus: 257mg; Carbohydrates: 7g; Fiber: 1g; Protein: 19g; Sugar: 3g

Thai-Style Chicken Stir-Fry

DIABETES-FRIENDLY, MEDIUM PROTEIN, ONE POT

Serves 4 • Prep time: 10 minutes • Cook time: 10 minutes

Fragrant Thai ingredients add great flavor to this easy stir-fry dish. Frozen stir-fry vegetables are the secret ingredient to this quick and convenient one-pot recipe. Use your favorite type or blend; just be sure to read labels to make sure that the vegetables aren't coated with a sauce.

¾ cup low-sodium chicken broth

1 tablespoon freshly squeezed lime juice

1 tablespoon cornstarch

2 teaspoons low-sodium soy sauce

1 teaspoon ground ginger

⅛ teaspoon red pepper flakes

2 tablespoons olive oil

12 ounces boneless skinless chicken breasts, cubed

2½ cups frozen stir-fry vegetables

¼ cup chopped unsalted roasted cashews

1. In a small bowl, whisk together the broth, lime juice, cornstarch, soy sauce, ginger, and red pepper flakes. Set aside.

2. Heat the olive oil in a wok or large skillet over medium-high heat.

3. Add the chicken and vegetables and stir-fry for 6 to 8 minutes or until the chicken reaches 165°F internal temperature and the vegetables are hot and tender-crisp.

4. Stir in the sauce and stir-fry for 1 to 2 minutes longer or until the sauce thickens and bubbles.

5. Sprinkle with the cashews and serve.

Make It Easier Tip: When purchasing chicken, or any type of meat, look for the label "all-natural." This label indicates that the meat is minimally processed, meaning that no chemical additives (such as phosphates) were added. Note that meats with the "all-natural" designation may still have added sodium. Check the nutrition label and look for meats with the lowest amount of sodium per serving.

Nutrition Info per Serving: Calories: 309; Total fat: 17g; Saturated fat: 3g; Sodium: 439mg; Potassium: 624mg; Phosphorus: 293mg; Carbohydrates: 16g; Fiber: 3g; Protein: 24g; Sugar: 6g

Vegetable and Turkey Kebabs

DIABETES-FRIENDLY, HIGH PROTEIN

Serves 4 • Prep time: 20 minutes • Cook time: 10 minutes

Turkey tenderloin is the perfect ingredient for making these kebabs. Lean and tender, it cuts easily into cubes and grills to juicy perfection. The addition of vegetables makes this recipe a meal. A savory garlic and mustard sauce is used to baste the kebabs as they grill, infusing the meat with flavor.

2 tablespoons olive oil

2 tablespoons freshly squeezed lemon juice

2 tablespoons yellow mustard

1 garlic clove, minced

1 teaspoon dried Italian seasoning

1 pound turkey tenderloin, cubed

16 whole small mushrooms

2 red bell peppers, cut into 1-inch pieces

1. Prepare and preheat the grill to medium coals and arrange the rack 6 inches from the heat.

2. In a small bowl, whisk together the olive oil, lemon juice, mustard, garlic, and Italian seasoning. Set aside.

3. Thread the turkey, mushrooms, and bell pepper onto 4 (10-inch) metal skewers, alternating meat and vegetables.

4. Place the kebabs on the rack and brush them with some of the olive oil mixture.

5. Close the grill and cook until the turkey reaches 165°F internal temperature, brushing twice with the olive oil mixture and turning the kebabs occasionally.

6. Brush the kebabs with all of the remaining marinade and cook, turning frequently, for 2 minutes longer. Serve.

Ingredient Tip: When a marinade is used to baste meat while it's cooking, the meat must be cooked for a minute after the final brushing to kill any bacteria. Dipping a brush into the marinade and onto raw meat will transfer bacteria to the marinade and the brush.

Nutrition Info per Serving: Calories: 225; Total fat: 9g; Saturated fat: 1g; Sodium: 218mg; Potassium: 557mg; Phosphorus: 288mg; Carbohydrates: 7g; Fiber: 2g; Protein: 29g; Sugar: 4g

Turkey Pho

DIABETES-FRIENDLY, MEDIUM PROTEIN

Serves 4 • Prep time: 10 minutes • Cook time: 20 minutes

Pho is a Vietnamese noodle soup that is usually made with leftover cooked meat such as turkey, chicken, or beef. Spices such as cloves and ginger add flavor and warmth to this simple and hearty dish, and the vegetables add color and texture. This is a great recipe to serve on a cold winter night.

1 tablespoon olive oil

½ pound ground white turkey meat

2 cups chopped Napa cabbage

1 large carrot, peeled and thinly sliced

3 scallions, white and green parts, chopped

2 garlic cloves, minced

1 teaspoon ground ginger

¼ teaspoon ground cloves

5 cups water

4 ounces dry rice noodles

1 tablespoon freshly squeezed lime juice

1. In a large pot, heat the oil over medium heat.

2. Add the ground turkey, cabbage, carrots, scallions, and garlic. Sauté for 4 to 5 minutes or until the turkey is browned.

3. Add the ginger, cloves, and water and bring to a simmer.

4. Reduce the heat to low and simmer 5 minutes.

5. Stir in the rice noodles and remove the pot from the heat; cover and let stand for 10 minutes or until the noodles are soft.

6. Stir in the lime juice and serve immediately.

Make It Easier Tip: You can omit the ground turkey and add 2 cups shredded leftover cooked turkey or chicken to this recipe; add it along with the noodles. You can also use pre-grated carrots instead of the sliced carrots to save a few minutes of prep time.

Increase Protein Tip: To make this high-protein, use ¾ pound turkey to increase the protein to 26 grams per serving.

Nutrition Info per Serving: Calories: 282; Total fat: 10g; Saturated fat: 2g; Sodium: 126mg; Potassium: 355mg; Phosphorus: 215mg; Carbohydrates: 29g; Fiber: 2g; Protein: 18g; Sugar: 3g

Turkey-Asparagus Risotto

HIGH PROTEIN

Serves 6 • Prep time: 10 minutes • Cook time: 20 minutes

Turkey and asparagus make a delicious combination. This simple risotto dish is pure comfort food and is simple to make. You do have to stand at the stove and stir the risotto pretty constantly while the rice is cooking, but it's worth it in the end. Serve in bowls along with some fresh fruit.

4 cups low-sodium chicken broth

2 tablespoons olive oil

1 onion, chopped

2 garlic cloves, minced

1 pound turkey tenderloin, cubed

1½ cups arborio rice or long-grain white rice

2 cups asparagus pieces

2 tablespoons unsalted butter

2 tablespoons grated Parmesan cheese

1. In a small saucepan over low heat, pour the broth and bring to a simmer.
2. Heat the oil in a large saucepan over medium heat.
3. Sauté the onion and garlic for 2 minutes.
4. Add the turkey and rice and sauté 2 more minutes.
5. Start adding the broth to the rice mixture, about ½ cup at a time, stirring constantly.
6. When the broth is absorbed, add more broth. You can stir less often as the rice begins to cook, but keep an eye on the pan.
7. After 15 minutes, add the asparagus to the rice mixture. Continue cooking and adding more broth.
8. The risotto is done when the rice is tender, and most of the broth is absorbed. This whole process should take about 20 minutes. You may not need all of the broth. This dish can be soupier or thicker, depending on how much broth you add and your taste.
9. Stir in the butter and cheese and serve immediately.

Reduce Protein Tip: To make this a medium-protein recipe, reduce the turkey to ¾ pound. The protein content will decrease to 22 grams per serving.

Nutrition Info per Serving: Calories: 380; Total fat: 11g; Saturated fat: 4g; Sodium: 175mg; Potassium: 498mg; Phosphorus: 297mg; Carbohydrates: 43g; Fiber: 2g; Protein: 26g; Sugar: 2g

Turkey Tenderloin with Berry Sauce

DIABETES-FRIENDLY, HIGH PROTEIN

Serves 4 • Prep time: 18 minutes • Cook time: 12 minutes

Sweet and tart berries are a great accent for juicy turkey meat. Think of traditional cranberry sauce as a reference. This recipe pairs nicely with a side of roasted vegetables. You could also make this dish with pork tenderloin. When you buy turkey at the store or butcher, make sure the product is not pre-seasoned.

2 tablespoons olive oil

1 pound turkey tenderloin, cut into 1-inch-thick slices

2 tablespoons all-purpose flour

Pinch salt

⅛ teaspoon freshly ground black pepper

1 cup sliced strawberries

1 cup raspberries

2 tablespoons strawberry jam

Juice from 1 lemon

2 tablespoons water

1. Heat the olive oil in a large skillet over medium heat.

2. Sprinkle the turkey slices with the flour, salt, and pepper.

3. Add the turkey to the skillet, cut-side down, and cook for 2 to 5 minutes per side, turning once, until it is lightly brown and registers 165°F internal temperature on a meat thermometer. "Cut-side down" means you put the side that touched the knife down in the pan. If you add the turkey to the skillet on the rounded side, it won't brown as well.

4. Transfer the turkey from the skillet to a clean plate and cover with foil to keep warm.

5. Add the strawberries, raspberries, jam, lemon juice, and water to the skillet. Mash the fruit with a potato masher.

6. Simmer the fruit mixture for 2 minutes.

7. Return the turkey to the skillet, stirring to coat with the berry sauce. Heat for 1 minute, then serve.

Nutrition Info per Serving: Calories: 261 Total fat: 9g; Saturated fat: 1g; Sodium: 171mg; Potassium: 403mg; Phosphorus: 252mg; Carbohydrates: 17g; Fiber: 3g; Protein: 28g; Sugar: 8g

Fiery Pork in Peanut Sauce

DIABETES-FRIENDLY, HIGH PROTEIN

Serves 6 • Prep time: 20 minutes • Cook time: 10 minutes

Pork tenderloin is another cut of meat that is sometimes overlooked for chicken or beef. This cut needs no preparation and is boneless, so just slice, cook, and serve it with savory and spicy peanut sauce. You can use this sauce on other meats, too; try it on halibut, turkey tenderloin, or chicken breasts.

⅓ cup crunchy peanut butter

½ cup low-sodium chicken broth

2 tablespoons freshly squeezed lemon juice

⅛ teaspoon red pepper flakes

2 tablespoons olive oil

1 pound pork tenderloin, cut into 1-inch slices

⅛ teaspoon cayenne pepper

1 onion, chopped

2 garlic cloves, minced

1 (8-ounce) package sliced mushrooms

⅓ cup grated carrots

1. In a small bowl, stir together the peanut butter, chicken broth, lemon juice, and red pepper flakes and set aside.

2. Heat the olive oil in a large skillet over medium heat.

3. Sprinkle the tenderloin slices with the cayenne pepper and place in the skillet.

4. Cook the pork, turning once, until it registers 145°F internal temperature. This should take 5 to 6 minutes in total.

5. Remove the pork from the skillet and set aside on a clean plate.

6. Add the onion, garlic, mushrooms, and carrot to the skillet. Sauté for 2 to 4 minutes or until tender-crisp.

7. Add the peanut sauce to the skillet and sauté for 1 minute. Then return the pork to the skillet and sauté for 1 to 2 minutes until heated through. Serve.

Ingredient Tip: When buying pork tenderloin, ask that it hasn't been injected with salt brine or seasoned in any manner.

Nutrition Info per Serving: Calories: 278; Total fat: 16g; Saturated fat: 4g; Sodium: 123mg; Potassium: 593mg; Phosphorus: 317mg; Carbohydrates: 8g; Fiber: 2g; Protein: 26g; Sugar: 4g

Lemon and Fruit Pork Kebabs

DIABETES-FRIENDLY, MEDIUM PROTEIN

Serves 4 • Prep time: 20 minutes • Cook time: 10 minutes

A plant-based diet prioritizes wholesome plant foods, like fruits and vegetables, at every meal. Most people think of fruit as more of a breakfast or snack food. This dinner recipe incorporates two types of fruit and pairs it with a small amount of pork. These sweet and sour kebabs taste great served alongside a tossed salad or roasted vegetable.

8 ounces boneless pork loin chops, cubed

1 cup canned pineapple chunks, drained, reserving ¼ cup juice

2 peaches, peeled and cubed

4 scallions, white and green parts, cut into 2-inch pieces

2 tablespoons olive oil

Juice of 1 lemon

2 tablespoons mustard

1 tablespoon cornstarch

2 teaspoons packed brown sugar

1. Prepare and preheat the grill to medium coals and set a grill 6 inches from the coals.

2. Thread the pork cubes, pineapple, peach cubes, and scallion pieces onto 4 (10-inch) metal skewers. Drizzle the kebabs with olive oil and set aside.

3. In a small saucepan, stir together the reserved pineapple juice, lemon juice, mustard, cornstarch, and brown sugar and bring to a simmer over medium heat. Simmer for 2 to 3 minutes or until the sauce boils and thickens. Remove from heat.

4. Place the kebabs on the grill. Grill for 8 to 10 minutes, turning frequently and brushing with the sauce until the pork registers at least 145°F internal temperature. Use all of the sauce.

5. Remove the kebabs from the heat and let stand for 5 minutes before serving.

Ingredient Tip: Pork can be cooked to medium-well and still be considered food safe. Cook it to at least 145°F, measured with a meat thermometer, and let the pork stand for 5 minutes. This wait time will raise the temperature to 150°F and maintain its juiciness.

Nutrition Info per Serving: Calories: 273; Total fat: 13g; Saturated fat: 3g; Sodium: 118mg; Potassium: 471mg; Phosphorus: 158mg; Carbohydrates: 22g; Fiber: 2g; Protein: 18g; Sugar: 17g

Beef and Bean Quesadillas

DIABETES-FRIENDLY, HIGH FIBER, MEDIUM PROTEIN

Serves 6 • Prep time: 10 minutes • Cook time: 20 minutes

This simple and delicious quesadilla recipe combines meat with flavorful veggies and savory cheese in a crisp tortilla. These layered sandwiches, which are nicely overstuffed, taste great topped with some Powerhouse Salsa (page 147). You could also serve the beef mixture over cooked brown rice instead of in the tortillas.

½ pound 85-percent-lean ground beef

1 onion, chopped

1 cup frozen corn, thawed and drained

½ cup low-sodium or no-salt-added canned black beans, drained and rinsed

2 teaspoons chili powder

¼ teaspoon garlic powder

6 (6-inch) corn tortillas

1 cup shredded Colby-Jack cheese

6 tablespoons sour cream

1. In a medium saucepan over medium heat, sauté the ground beef and onion until the meat is browned and cooked through, 5 to 7 minutes. Remove the pan from the heat and drain off the excess fat.

2. Stir in the corn, beans, chili powder, and garlic powder into the meat mixture.

3. Place the tortillas on your work surface. Divide the beef mixture among half of the tortillas, spreading it out to about ½-inch from the edges. Top with the cheese and the remaining tortillas.

4. Place a large skillet over medium-high heat. Add the quesadillas one at a time. Cook for 2 to 3 minutes on each side, turning once, until the tortillas are crisp.

5. Repeat until all are cooked.

6. Cut each quesadilla into fourths with a sharp butcher knife and serve with the sour cream.

Increase Protein Tip: To make this a high-protein recipe, use 1 pound of the lean ground beef. The protein content will increase to 29 grams per serving.

Nutrition Info per ½ Quesadilla: Calories: 288; Total fat: 15g; Saturated fat: 5g; Sodium: 316mg; Potassium: 366 mg; Phosphorus: 274mg; Carbohydrates: 33g; Fiber: 6g; Protein: 18g; Sugar: 2g

Steak Stir-Fry

DIABETES-FRIENDLY, LOW PROTEIN

Serves 4 • Prep time: 20 minutes • Cook time: 10 minutes

Stir-fry recipes are a great dinner choice because you get to enjoy the satisfying taste and texture of meat while eating a dinner composed mostly of vegetables. This recipe's meat is tender and silky because of a technique called velveting, where it's coated in a mixture of cornstarch and baking soda so that it retains its juices while cooking. Prepare all of your ingredients before you start cooking since there won't be time to stop and chop during the cooking process. This recipe pairs deliciously with rice noodles or rice.

8 ounces top sirloin steak, cubed

3 tablespoons cornstarch, divided

½ teaspoon baking soda

1 cup low-sodium beef broth

2 teaspoons hoisin sauce

½ teaspoon ground ginger

⅛ teaspoon freshly ground black pepper

2 tablespoons olive oil

1 onion, chopped

2 garlic cloves, minced

1 red bell pepper, chopped

1 cup snow peas

1. In a medium bowl, toss the steak cubes with 1 tablespoon cornstarch and the baking soda to thoroughly coat. Let this mixture stand while you prepare the rest of the ingredients.

2. In a small bowl, stir together the beef broth, remaining 2 tablespoons cornstarch, hoisin sauce, ginger, and pepper. Set aside.

3. Heat the oil in a large wok or skillet over medium-high heat.

4. Stir-fry the beef for 2 minutes or until it starts to brown.

5. Transfer the beef to a clean plate with a slotted spoon and set aside.

6. Add the onion and garlic to the skillet and stir-fry for 2 minutes. Add the red bell pepper and snow peas and stir-fry 2 minutes longer.

7. Return the beef to the skillet and pour in the sauce.

8. Stir-fry for 2 to 3 minutes longer or until the steak is 145°F internal temperature and the sauce bubbles and thickens. Serve.

Nutrition Info per Serving: Calories: 198; Total fat: 10g; Saturated fat: 2g; Sodium: 271mg; Potassium: 372mg; Phosphorus: 153mg; Carbohydrates: 13g; Fiber: 2g; Protein: 14g; Sugar: 4g

Beef and Mushroom Meatballs

DIABETES-FRIENDLY, MEDIUM PROTEIN

Serves 4 • Prep time: 15 minutes • Cook time: 15 minutes

These meatballs are extra nutritious and juicy thanks to the addition of finely chopped mushrooms to the lean ground beef. These meatballs pair nicely with a side of vegetables, such as Sautéed Spicy Cabbage (page 42). For a convenient make-ahead meal, double this batch and freeze half up to 2 months. To use, let the meatballs thaw overnight in the refrigerator and add them to soups or pasta.

1 recipe Duxelles (page 144)

8 ounces 85-percent-lean ground beef

2 tablespoons crushed puffed rice cereal

1 large egg

1 teaspoon dried Italian seasoning

Pinch salt

⅛ teaspoon freshly ground black pepper

2 tablespoons olive oil

1. Mix together the Duxelles, beef, crushed puffed rice cereal, egg, Italian seasoning, salt, and pepper in a large bowl until thoroughly combined.

2. Form the mixture into 24 meatballs.

3. Heat the olive oil in a large skillet over medium-high heat and add the meatballs.

4. Cook, turning occasionally, until the meatballs are browned and cooked through to 165°F internal temperature, 14 to 17 minutes.

5. Serve.

Increase Protein Tip: To make this a high-protein recipe, increase the ground beef to ¾ pound and the crushed rice cereal to ⅓ cup. The protein content will increase to 25 grams per serving.

Nutrition Info per 6 Meatballs: Calories: 292; Total fat: 23g; Saturated fat: 7g; Sodium: 116mg; Potassium: 465mg; Phosphorus: 203mg; Carbohydrates: 5g; Fiber: 1g; Protein: 18g; Sugar: 2g

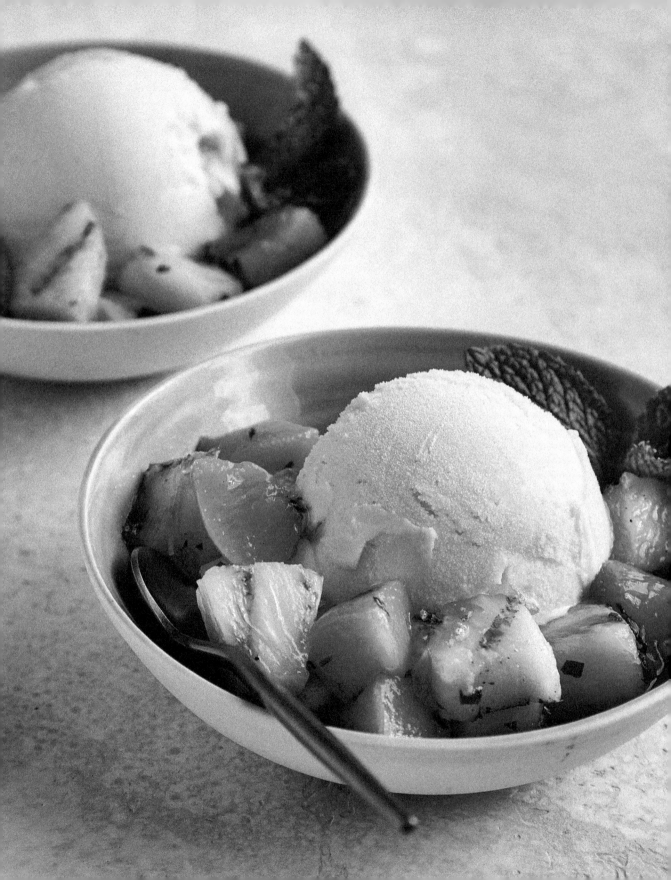

7

Sweet Treats and Snacks

⇐ *Grilled Pineapple and Peach Mint Sundaes, page 137*

Berries with Warm Vanilla Sauce

HIGH FIBER, MEDIUM PROTEIN

Serves 4 • Prep time: 15 minutes • Cook time: 10 minutes

Fresh mixed berries topped with a warm vanilla-infused sauce are a delicious dessert you can make in minutes. This recipe includes only a small amount of milk per serving, which helps limit the total phosphorus content of the dish.

½ vanilla bean

1 cup 2-percent milk

3 tablespoons
granulated sugar

1 tablespoon
all-purpose flour

1 large egg

½ teaspoon
vanilla extract

1 cup raspberries

1 cup sliced strawberries

1 cup blueberries

1. Cut the vanilla bean in half lengthwise and scrape out the seeds with the side of a sharp knife. Store the remaining half bean wrapped in plastic for another recipe.

2. In a small nonreactive saucepan, stir together the milk, vanilla seeds, and the vanilla bean over medium heat until steaming, about 3 minutes.

3. Meanwhile, whisk together the sugar, flour, and egg in a small bowl.

4. Remove the vanilla bean from the milk and discard. Gradually whisk ¼ cup of the warm milk into the egg mixture in the bowl until smooth.

5. Add the egg mixture to the milk in the saucepan and cook over medium-low heat, stirring frequently, until thickened, 4 to 5 minutes.

6. Remove the pan from the heat and stir in the vanilla extract. Place the whole pan into a large bowl filled with ice to cool a bit while you prepare the berries.

7. Divide the raspberries, strawberries, and blueberries among four bowls.

8. Stir the cooled sauce with the whisk and divide it among the berries. Serve immediately.

Diabetes Tip: Replacing the sugar in this recipe with powdered erythritol will lower the sugar content to 10g per serving.

Nutrition Info per Serving: Calories: 145; Total fat: 3g; Saturated fat: 1g; Sodium: 45mg; Potassium: 238mg; Phosphorus: 102mg; Carbohydrates: 26g; Fiber: 4g; Protein: 5g; Sugar: 20g

Apple Pie Sundaes

HIGH FIBER, MEDIUM PROTEIN

Serves 4 • Prep time: 10 minutes • Cook time: 10 minutes

This delectable sundae is dressed up with some crushed cookies and sweet butter-sautéed apples. It tastes like an apple pie without all the hassle. Vanilla wafers and chopped pecans make up the "crust" in the sundae, which adds satisfying texture to this effortless dessert recipe.

1 tablespoon
  unsalted butter
2 Granny Smith apples,
  cored and chopped
1 tablespoon freshly
  squeezed lemon juice

1 tablespoon packed
  brown sugar
1 teaspoon cinnamon
½ cup crushed
  vanilla wafers

2 tablespoons
  chopped pecans
2 cups vanilla
  whole-milk yogurt

1. In a large skillet, melt the butter over medium heat.

2. Add the apples; sprinkle with the lemon juice, brown sugar, and cinnamon, and stir.

3. Sauté the apples, stirring frequently, for 10 to 12 minutes or until the apples are tender. Transfer the apple mixture from the skillet to a medium bowl.

4. In a small bowl, stir together the wafers and pecans.

5. Evenly divide the yogurt between four dessert cups. Top each with the apple mixture and the pecan mixture and serve immediately.

Ingredient Tip: You can choose any type of apple you'd like in this recipe. Apples that are good for cooking include Granny Smith, Honeycrisp, Jonathan, Winesap, or Cortland.

Diabetes Tip: To make this a diabetes-friendly recipe, replace vanilla yogurt with plain yogurt. Eliminate the brown sugar and replace with 2 tablespoons of powdered erythritol (or more to taste). Instead of using the vanilla wafers, add an extra tablespoon of chopped pecans. The sugar content will decrease to 14g per serving, and the carbohydrate content will decrease to 19g per serving.

Nutrition Info per Serving: Calories: 274; Total fat: 11g; Saturated fat: 5g; Sodium: 89mg; Potassium: 353mg; Phosphorus: 135mg; Carbohydrates: 39g; Fiber: 3g; Protein: 5g; Sugar: 31g

Berry Frozen Yogurt Tartlets

HIGH FIBER, LOW PROTEIN

Serves 6 • Prep time: 15 minutes

Dessert is an exceptional treat that one should always savor and enjoy. This decadent dessert also happens to be a good source of fiber, thanks to the inclusion of colorful and flavorful berries and nutty pecans. Use your favorite frozen vanilla yogurt as the creamy base for this recipe.

9 whole graham crackers, crushed (about ⅔ cup)

2 tablespoons brown sugar

2 tablespoons crushed pecans

3 tablespoons unsalted butter, melted

½ cup mashed strawberries

½ cup raspberries

½ cup blueberries

2 cups regular vanilla frozen yogurt

1. Line 6 muffin tins with paper liners.

2. In a medium bowl, stir together the graham cracker crumbs, brown sugar, pecans, and butter to form coarse crumbs.

3. Press the crumb mixture into the muffin tins to create tart cups and place in the freezer while you prepare the berries.

4. In a small bowl, gently stir together the strawberries, raspberries, and blueberries.

5. Scoop the frozen yogurt into the prepared cups and top with the berry mixture. Serve.

Make It Easier Tip: Purchasing pre-crumbled graham cracker crumbs will save you some time prepping.

Nutrition Info per Serving: Calories: 213; Total fat: 10g; Saturated fat: 5g; Sodium: 81mg; Potassium: 191mg; Phosphorus: 88mg; Carbohydrates: 29g; Fiber: 3g; Protein: 3g; Sugar: 20g

Instant Peach Melba Sorbet

5-INGREDIENT, HIGH FIBER, LOW PROTEIN

Serves 4 • Prep time: 15 minutes • Cook time: 10 minutes

This recipe for instant sorbet is somewhat like a smoothie, but much richer in fruit so it is firm and ready to eat as soon as it's blended. You will need a powerful food processor or blender to make this recipe because the frozen fruit can be very hard. If you make this dessert ahead, transfer it to a loaf pan, cover, and freeze up to 3 days. Let the sorbet stand at room temperature for 10 minutes before serving, so it's easier to scoop.

2 cups frozen peach slices	½ cup plain whole-milk yogurt	1 teaspoon vanilla
1 cup frozen raspberries	1 tablespoon honey	

1. Combine the peaches, raspberries, yogurt, honey, and vanilla in a food processor or blender. Process or blend until the mixture is smooth; this will take a few minutes. Put a towel over the processor to help muffle the noise.

2. Serve immediately or cover and freeze for a few hours before serving.

Diabetes Tip: To make this a diabetes-friendly recipe, replace the honey with 1 to 2 tablespoons of powdered erythritol. The sugar content will decrease to 10g per serving.

Nutrition Info per Serving: Calories: 100; Total fat: 1g; Saturated fat: less than 1g; Sodium: 19mg; Potassium: 270mg; Phosphorus: 60mg; Carbohydrates: 21g; Fiber: 6g; Protein: 2g; Sugar: 15g

Thyme and Pineapple Crisp

HIGH FIBER, LOW PROTEIN

Serves 6 • Prep time: 15 minutes • Cook time: 10 minutes

A crisp is a dessert made with some kind of fruit base and a crunchy topping with oats and brown sugar. Ordinarily, a crisp would need a minimum of an hour in the oven, but this version cuts that time by sautéing the pineapple in a saucepan and making the topping separately in a skillet.

1 (20-ounce) can pineapple tidbits in juice, drained, reserving ⅓ cup juice

¼ cup brown sugar, divided

1 tablespoon cornstarch

½ teaspoon dried thyme leaves

3 tablespoons unsalted butter

1¼ cups quick-cooking oats

⅓ cup whole-wheat flour

Pinch salt

2 tablespoons chopped walnuts

1. Stir together the drained pineapple, reserved pineapple juice, 1 tablespoon brown sugar, cornstarch, and the thyme leaves in a medium saucepan over medium heat.

2. Cook for 8 to 10 minutes, stirring occasionally, until the mixture is thickened.

3. Meanwhile, combine the remaining 3 tablespoons brown sugar and butter in a medium skillet over medium heat, stirring frequently, until the mixture melts.

4. Add the oats, flour, salt, and walnuts to the brown sugar mixture in the skillet.

5. Cook, stirring frequently, until the mixture is a deep golden brown, about 5 minutes. Transfer the oat mixture to a plate.

6. When the pineapple mixture is thickened, top with the oatmeal mixture right in the saucepan and serve.

Ingredient Tip: You can use pineapple chunks or even crushed pineapple in this recipe. Just be sure to drain it well before you start. Choose pineapple that is canned in juice, not syrup, or the sugar content will be much higher.

Nutrition Info per Serving: Calories: 238; Total fat: 9g; Saturated fat: 4g; Sodium: 31mg; Potassium: 221mg; Phosphorus: 109mg; Carbohydrates: 39g; Fiber: 3g; Protein: 4g; Sugar: 20g

Big Peanut Butter Macadamia Cookie

HIGH FIBER, MEDIUM PROTEIN

Serves 4 • Prep time: 15 minutes • Cook time: 15 minutes

How fun is it to make one big cookie and let everyone break off a piece? You will feel like you are at a party! This cookie is much faster to make than individual smaller cookies and is delicious served warm. The buttery macadamia nuts are used instead of chopped peanuts to reduce the potassium content of this recipe.

2 tablespoons unsalted butter	1 large egg	¼ teaspoon Low Phosphorus Baking Powder (page 140)
3 tablespoons peanut butter	1 large egg yolk	
⅓ cup brown sugar	½ teaspoon vanilla	2 tablespoons chopped macadamia nuts
	⅓ cup all-purpose flour	
	⅓ cup whole-wheat flour	

1. Preheat the oven to 350°F. Line a baking sheet with parchment paper and set aside.

2. In a medium microwave-safe bowl, melt the butter on high power for 30 seconds.

3. Stir in the peanut butter, brown sugar, egg, egg yolk, and vanilla until smooth.

4. Add the all-purpose flour, whole-wheat flour, and baking powder and mix until just combined.

5. Form the dough into a 5-inch round on the parchment paper and sprinkle with the macadamia nuts.

6. Bake for 14 to16 minutes or until the cookie is set and light golden brown. Serve warm.

Ingredient Tip: To reduce the sodium in this recipe to 52 milligrams, you can use unsalted peanut butter.

Diabetes Tip: To make this recipe diabetes-friendly, replace the sugar with ⅓ cup plus 1 tablespoon of powdered erythritol. The sugar content will decrease to 2g per serving.

Nutrition Info per Serving: Calories: 323; Total fat: 17g; Saturated fat: 6g; Sodium: 171mg; Potassium: 249mg; Phosphorus: 134mg; Carbohydrates: 36g; Fiber: 2g; Protein: 8g; Sugar: 19g

Chocolate Cheesecake Bites

LOW PROTEIN

Serves 6 • Prep time: 30 minutes

There's no need to exclude chocolate completely from your renal diet. Like many foods, it's about moderation. A small number of chocolate chips lend a delicious flavor to this easy, no-bake recipe. Make sure you use semisweet or dark chocolate to keep the sugar content lower. You can store these in the refrigerator for up to two days.

½ cup vanilla
    wafer crumbs
3 tablespoons
    unsalted butter

½ cup semisweet
    chocolate
    chips, divided
4 ounces cream
    cheese, softened

2 tablespoons
    sour cream
¼ cup powdered sugar
½ teaspoon vanilla

1. In a small bowl, stir together the wafer crumbs and butter until well mixed.

2. Divide this mixture among 12 mini muffin cups and press the crumbs firmly into the bottom of each cup. Refrigerate while you prepare the filling.

3. Melt the chocolate chips in a small microwave-safe bowl for 1 minute on high power, stirring after 30 seconds. Remove and reserve 2 tablespoons of the melted chocolate.

4. In a medium bowl, beat the cream cheese with the sour cream with electric hand beaters until smooth.

5. Add the powdered sugar and vanilla and beat until combined, scraping down the sides of the bowl with a spatula.

6. Add the melted chocolate and beat until smooth.

7. Divide the cream cheese mixture among the muffin cups evenly and drizzle with the reserved chocolate. Serve.

Make It Easier Tip: You can make these mini cheesecakes ahead of time. Cover and chill for 2 to 3 hours before serving.

Nutrition Info per 2 Cheesecakes: Calories: 250; Total fat: 19g; Saturated fat: 11g; Sodium: 85mg; Potassium: 95mg; Phosphorus: 52mg; Carbohydrates: 21g; Fiber: 1g; Protein: 2g; Sugar: 17g

Grilled Pineapple and Peach Mint Sundaes

5-INGREDIENT, HIGH FIBER, LOW PROTEIN

Serves 4 • Prep time: 20 minutes • Cook time: 10 minutes

Grilling fruit caramelizes the sugar, adding wonderful rich flavor and color to any recipe. Pouring warm fruit over ice cream creates a delicious contrast in texture and temperature. If you want to use a fresh pineapple, remove the skin and core and slice the pineapple into spears.

4 pineapple slices, canned in juice, drained

4 peach halves, canned in juice, drained

1 tablespoon chopped fresh mint

2 tablespoons peach jam

2 cups regular vanilla frozen yogurt

1. Prepare and preheat the grill to medium. Place a clean grill rack 6 inches from the coals.

2. Pat the pineapples and peaches dry with a clean kitchen towel.

3. Put the fruit on the grill and grill for 2 minutes per side, turning once, until the fruit has nice grill marks.

4. Cut the fruit into bite-size pieces and place in a bowl. Stir in the mint and the peach jam.

5. Divide the frozen yogurt among four dessert cups and top with the fruit mixture. Serve immediately.

Make It Easier Tip: You can use a grill pan placed on your stovetop instead of using an outdoor grill for this recipe. Place the pan on the stovetop and heat over high heat for 3 minutes. Reduce the heat to medium and add the fruit. Or if using a portable indoor grill; heat according to manufacturer's instructions.

Nutrition Info per Serving: Calories: 200; Total fat: 3g; Saturated fat: 2g; Sodium: 62mg; Potassium: 309mg; Phosphorus: 98mg; Carbohydrates: 42g; Fiber: 2g; Protein: 3g; Sugar: 37g

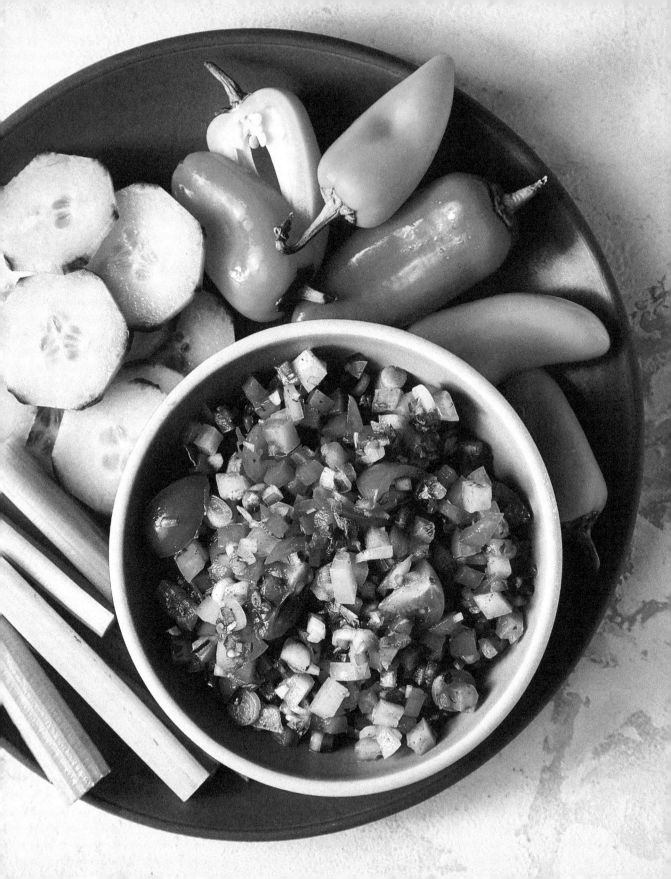

8

Broths, Condiments, and Seasoning Mixes

⇐*Powerhouse Salsa, page 147*

Low Phosphorus Baking Powder

5-INGREDIENT, DIABETES-FRIENDLY, LOW PROTEIN

Makes 10 tablespoons • Prep time: 20 minutes

Baking powder is very high in phosphorus. Luckily, you can make a low-phosphorus version yourself using just three ingredients. Baking powder is made of alkaline and acidic components. When combined with liquid, they produce carbon dioxide, which makes baked goods rise. Since this ingredient is usually used in small amounts, the amount of potassium per serving is very low.

6 tablespoons cream of tartar

3 tablespoons baking soda

1 tablespoon cornstarch

1. Combine the cream of tartar, baking soda, and cornstarch in a small bowl and whisk to combine.
2. Force the mixture through a fine sieve to remove any lumps.
3. Store in an airtight container at room temperature and use in baking recipes.

Ingredient Tip: Most commercial baking powder is double-acting, which means it produces CO_2 when it gets wet and again in the heat of the oven. In single-acting baking powder like this one, the CO_2 is only produced when liquid is introduced. To get the best results with this powder, make sure to put the batter or dough into the oven as quickly as possible.

Nutrition Info per 1 Teaspoon: Calories: 6; Total fat: 0; Saturated fat: 2g; Sodium: 379mg; Potassium: 297mg; Phosphorus: 0mg; Carbohydrates: 1g; Fiber: 0g; Protein: 0g; Sugar: 0g

Everyday No-Salt Seasoning Blend

DIABETES-FRIENDLY, LOW PROTEIN

Makes 2 tablespoons • Prep time: 10 minutes

This recipe can also be made from your favorite dried herbs and spices. Just keep to the general proportions in this recipe and experiment until you find your favorite blend. Be sure to write down the ingredients when you make one you like so you can reproduce it. You can keep this on your dining room table in a shaker and add it to your meals whenever you want.

1 teaspoon dried thyme leaves

1 teaspoon dried marjoram leaves

1 teaspoon dried basil leaves

1 teaspoon dried oregano leaves

½ teaspoon onion powder

½ teaspoon garlic powder

½ teaspoon ground mustard

¼ teaspoon freshly ground black pepper

¼ teaspoon paprika

Combine the thyme, marjoram, basil, oregano, onion powder, garlic powder, ground mustard, pepper, and paprika and keep in a small jar with a tight lid at room temperature for up to 6 months.

Ingredient Tip: Try savory, sage, dill weed, dried parsley, tarragon, celery seed, dill seed, fennel seed, or ground ginger for different flavor profiles.

Nutrition Info per 1 Teaspoon: Calories: 4; Total fat: 0g; Saturated fat: 0g; Sodium: 1mg; Potassium: 17mg; Phosphorus: 4mg; Carbohydrates: 1g; Fiber: 0g; Protein: 0g; Sugar: 0g

Thai-Style Seasoning Blend

DIABETES-FRIENDLY, LOW PROTEIN

Makes 3 tablespoons • Prep time: 10 minutes

This fragrant and flavorful seasoning blend is delicious as a rub for fish, chicken, or even pork. It's also good sprinkled into soups or salads or on roasted vegetables. Also, try it in your favorite vinaigrette or dip. The combination of ingredients, especially the mint, ginger, and cumin, are common in Thai cuisine.

1½ teaspoons turmeric

1½ teaspoons paprika

1 teaspoon
   ground coriander

1 teaspoon
   ground ginger

1 teaspoon dry mustard

1 teaspoon ground cumin

1 teaspoon dried mint
   leaves, crushed

1 teaspoon red
   pepper flakes

Combine the turmeric, paprika, coriander, ginger, dry mustard, cumin, mint, and red pepper flakes and keep in a small jar with a tight lid at room temperature for up to 6 months.

Ingredient Tip: This blend can be adjusted to your preferred level of spiciness. For a milder blend, decrease or eliminate the red pepper flakes. For a spicier flavor, increase the red pepper flakes to 1½ teaspoons or add some cayenne pepper.

Nutrition Info per 1 Teaspoon: Calories: 5; Total fat: 0g; Saturated fat: 0g; Sodium: 1mg; Potassium: 30mg; Phosphorus: 6mg; Carbohydrates: 1g; Fiber: 0g; Protein: 0g; Sugar: 0g

Tex-Mex Seasoning Mix

DIABETES-FRIENDLY, LOW PROTEIN

Makes 2 tablespoons • Prep time: 10 minutes

This spicy seasoning mix is wonderful on roasted vegetables or as an ingredient for your favorite Tex-Mex dish. You can make this mix spicier by adding more cayenne pepper or crushed red pepper flakes. Use it in burritos or quesadillas, or add to any dip recipe for a southwest flair.

1 tablespoon chili powder

½ teaspoon ground cumin

½ teaspoon dried oregano leaves

½ teaspoon garlic powder

½ teaspoon onion powder

½ teaspoon cayenne pepper

½ teaspoon red pepper flakes

Combine the chili powder, cumin, oregano, garlic powder, onion powder, cayenne pepper, and red pepper flakes and keep in a small jar with a tight lid at room temperature for up to 6 months.

Ingredient Tip: For a milder seasoning mix, omit the cayenne pepper and decrease the red pepper flakes to ⅛ teaspoon.

Nutrition Info per 1 Teaspoon: Calories: 7; Total fat: 0g; Saturated fat: 0g; Sodium: 39mg; Potassium: 38mg; Phosphorus: 7mg; Carbohydrates: 1g; Fiber: 1g; Protein: 0g; Sugar: 0g

Duxelles

Serves 8 • Prep time: 15 minutes • Cook time: 15 minutes

This recipe may sound fancy, but it's just sautéed mushrooms with garlic and scallions. The mushrooms are chopped very fine and sautéed until brown, so they become very flavorful. You can add duxelles to soups or sauces for a wonderful meaty flavor, or use them to top grilled chicken or pork. They are the secret ingredient in the Beef and Mushroom Meatballs (page 126).

1 (8-ounce)
   package sliced
   cremini mushrooms
3 scallions, white and
   green parts

3 garlic cloves
1 tablespoon olive oil
1 tablespoon
   unsalted butter

1 teaspoon freshly
   squeezed lemon juice
Pinch salt

1. Finely chop the mushrooms, scallions, and garlic in a food processor or blender.

2. Place the mushroom mixture in the middle of a kitchen towel, gather up the ends to create a pouch, and squeeze the pouch over the sink to remove some of the liquid in the mushrooms.

3. Heat the olive oil and butter in a large skillet over medium-high heat.

4. Add the drained mushroom mixture to the skillet and sprinkle with the lemon juice and salt.

5. Sauté for 8 to 12 minutes, stirring frequently, or until the mushrooms are browned.

6. This mixture can be refrigerated up to 4 days or frozen up to 1 month.

Ingredient Tip: You can use button mushrooms for this recipe if you can't find cremini mushrooms. The recipe will be just as flavorful and less expensive.

Nutrition Info per 2-Tablespoon Serving: Calories: 37; Total fat: 3g; Saturated fat: 1g; Sodium: 22mg; Potassium: 141mg; Phosphorus: 37mg; Carbohydrates: 2g; Fiber: 0g; Protein: 1g; Sugar: 1g

Chicken Stock

DIABETES-FRIENDLY, LOW PROTEIN

Makes 4 cups • Prep time: 5 minutes • Cook time: 25 minutes

Homemade chicken broth in 30 minutes seems improbable, but it can be done. If you want a richer-tasting broth, simmer the ingredients for 2 to 3 hours. However, this quick version is better than anything you can buy from a store, so make a batch or two and store in the freezer in convenient 1 cup portions.

1 tablespoon olive oil

1 bone-in skin-on chicken breast (3 to 4 ounces)

Pinch salt

1 onion, unpeeled, sliced

1 carrot, unpeeled, sliced

1 bay leaf

5 cups water

1. Heat the olive oil in a large saucepan over medium-high heat.

2. Sprinkle the chicken with salt and add to the pan, skin-side down. Brown for 2 minutes.

3. Add the onion and carrot and cook for 1 minute longer.

4. Add the bay leaf and water and bring to a boil.

5. Reduce the heat to medium-low and simmer for 20 to 22 minutes, stirring occasionally. Skim off and discard any scum that rises to the surface.

6. Strain the stock through a fine-mesh colander into a bowl. You can reserve the chicken breast for other recipes, although it may be tough after cooking. Discard the remaining solids.

7. Refrigerate the broth and skim off any fat that rises to the top. You can freeze this stock in 1-cup measures to use in recipes.

8. Store in the refrigerator up to 3 days; freeze up to 3 months.

Ingredient tip: Did you know that broth made with bone-in meat is called stock? Using bone-in chicken makes the liquid taste richer.

Nutrition Info per ½-Cup Serving: Calories: 37; Total fat: 2g; Saturated fat: 0g; Sodium: 22mg; Potassium: 85mg; Phosphorus: 30mg; Carbohydrates: 2g; Fiber: 0g; Protein: 3g; Sugar: 1g

Vegetable Broth

DIABETES-FRIENDLY, LOW PROTEIN

Makes 4 cups • Prep time: 20 minutes

Vegetable broth is an essential ingredient in many of these recipes. Making your own is easy and adds much more flavor to any recipe than just using plain water. Don't skip the browning step; that is the trick for adding rich veggie taste to the finished broth. Get the vegetables nice and brown for best results.

1 tablespoon olive oil

1 unpeeled onion, sliced

2 unpeeled garlic
  cloves, crushed

2 unpeeled carrots,
  sliced

2 celery stalks, cut into
  2-inch pieces

1 bay leaf

1 teaspoon dried
  basil leaves

5 cups water

1. Heat the olive oil in a large saucepan over medium-high heat.

2. Sauté the onion, garlic, carrot, and celery for 5 minutes, stirring frequently, or until lightly browned.

3. Add the bay leaf, basil, and water to the saucepan and bring to a boil.

4. Reduce the heat to medium-low and simmer for 20 to 22 minutes, stirring occasionally. Skim off and discard any scum that rises to the surface.

5. Strain the stock through a fine-mesh colander into a bowl. Discard the solids.

6. Refrigerate the broth and remove any fat that rises to the top. You can freeze this broth in 1-cup measures to use in recipes.

7. Store in the refrigerator up to 3 days; freeze up to 3 months.

Ingredient Tip: Always remove bay leaves from recipes before you eat. The center spine of the bay leaf is sharp and can hurt your esophagus if you eat it.

Nutrition Info per ½-Cup Serving: Calories: 31; Total fat: 2g; Saturated fat: 0g; Sodium: 21mg; Potassium: 110mg; Phosphorus: 14mg; Carbohydrates: 4g; Fiber: 1g; Protein: 0g; Sugar: 2g

Powerhouse Salsa

DIABETES-FRIENDLY, HIGH FIBER, LOW PROTEIN, ONE POT

Serves 8 • Prep time: 20 minutes

Most salsas are made with tomatoes, tomato purée, and lots of salt. As a result, the potassium and sodium content can really add up. This salsa is spicy and colorful, made with just a small amount of grape tomatoes for color. Use it in recipes in this book or as a dip for fruits and veggies.

8 grape tomatoes, chopped

1 yellow bell pepper, chopped

1 red bell pepper, chopped

¼ cup minced red onion

3 scallions, white and green parts, chopped

1 garlic clove, minced

1 jalapeño pepper, minced

2 tablespoons chopped fresh cilantro

2 teaspoons chili powder

2 tablespoons freshly squeezed lime juice

Combine the tomatoes, yellow bell pepper, red bell pepper, red onion, scallions, garlic, jalapeño, cilantro, chili powder, and lime juice in a medium bowl and mix. Use immediately or cover and store in the refrigerator up to 4 days.

Make It Easier Tip: You can freeze salsa for up to three months. Thaw the salsa in the refrigerator and pour out any excess liquid before using it.

Nutrition Info per 2-Tablespoon Serving: Calories: 20; Total fat: 0g; Saturated fat: 0g; Sodium: 22mg; Potassium: 148mg; Phosphorus: 19mg; Carbohydrates: 5g; Fiber: 2g; Protein: 1g; Sugar: 3g

Pesto

DIABETES-FRIENDLY, LOW PROTEIN

Serves 16 • Prep time: 15 minutes

Pesto is a flavorful Italian no-cook sauce that is made from fresh basil, garlic, pine nuts, and olive oil. It can be used in so many ways, such as an addition to salad dressing, a sauce for pasta, and even as a sandwich spread. You must use fresh basil in this recipe for the best taste and color. This fragrant herb is readily available in grocery stores in the produce section.

2 cups fresh basil leaves
½ cup flat-leaf parsley
2 garlic cloves, sliced
3 tablespoons olive oil,
   plus more for drizzling

2 tablespoons grated
   Parmesan cheese
2 tablespoons
   chopped walnuts
2 tablespoons water

1 tablespoon freshly
   squeezed lemon juice

1. Combine the basil, parsley, garlic, olive oil, cheese, walnuts, water, and lemon juice in a blender or food processor and blend or process until the mixture is almost smooth.

2. You can also use a mortar and pestle to grind all of the ingredients together.

3. Put the pesto in a small bowl and drizzle more olive oil on top to prevent browning. Store in the refrigerator up to 3 days.

Make It Easier Tip: This pesto freezes beautifully. Just spoon the pesto into plastic ice cube trays and freeze until firm. Pop the cubes out of the tray, put them into a freezer bag, and store in the freezer up to 3 months. To use, thaw the pesto cubes in the refrigerator before you add them to a recipe. Or just drop a cube into a pasta sauce or soup and let it cook.

Nutrition Info per 2-Tablespoon Serving: Calories: 34; Total fat: 3g; Saturated fat: 1g; Sodium: 16mg; Potassium: 35mg; Phosphorus: 13mg; Carbohydrates: 1g; Fiber: 0g; Protein: 1g; Sugar: 0g

Ranch Seasoning Mix

DIABETES-FRIENDLY, LOW PROTEIN

Makes ⅓ cup • Prep time: 10 minutes

Ranch salad dressing is made from buttermilk and lots of different types of herbs and spices. You can use this delicious mix to season salads, vegetables, and to sprinkle on meats such as beef, chicken, fish, and pork. Or use it to make a dip by combining it with some cream cheese and then spreading on crackers as a snack.

2 tablespoons dried
   buttermilk powder

1 tablespoon cornstarch

1 tablespoon
   dried parsley

1 teaspoon dried
   dill weed

1 teaspoon dried chives

½ teaspoon
   garlic powder

½ teaspoon
   onion powder

¼ teaspoon freshly
   ground black pepper

Combine the buttermilk powder, cornstarch, parsley, dill weed, chives, garlic powder, onion powder, and pepper and keep in a small jar with a tight lid at room temperature for up to 6 months.

Ingredient Tip: To make a dip with this recipe, combine ¼ cup whole-milk plain yogurt with 2 tablespoons sour cream, 1 tablespoon unsweetened almond milk, and 2 teaspoons of this seasoning mix. Serve with fresh vegetables.

Nutrition Info per 1 Teaspoon: Calories: 8; Total fat: less than 1g; Saturated fat: less than 1g; Sodium: 1mg; Potassium: 27mg; Phosphorus: 4mg; Carbohydrates: 1g; Fiber: less than 1g; Protein: less than 1g; Sugar: less than 1g

Poultry Seasoning Mix

DIABETES-FRIENDLY, LOW PROTEIN

Makes 2 tablespoons • Prep time: 20 minutes

This delicious and savory combination of ingredients is a classic culinary blend. Although this recipe is "poultry" seasoning mix, you can use it on any meat, such as beef or pork, and even on roasted vegetables or in a salad dressing for extra flavor.

2 teaspoons dried
thyme leaves

2 teaspoons dried
basil leaves

1½ teaspoons dried
marjoram leaves

¼ teaspoon
onion powder

¼ teaspoon
garlic powder

⅛ teaspoon freshly
ground black pepper

1. Combine the thyme, basil, marjoram, onion powder, garlic powder, and pepper in a small bowl and mix. Store in a small jar with a tight-fitting lid at room temperature.

2. You can grind all of these ingredients together to make a mixture that is more like commercial poultry seasoning.

Ingredient Tip: Use your favorite herbs in this easy recipe. You might want to add sage or reduce the amount of basil.

Nutrition Info per ½-Teaspoon Serving: Calories: 21; Total fat: less than 1g; Saturated fat: 2g; Sodium: 23mg; Potassium: 132mg; Phosphorus: 17mg; Carbohydrates: 5g; Fiber: 2g; Protein: 1g; Sugar: 3g

Homemade Mustard

DIABETES-FRIENDLY, LOW PROTEIN, ONE POT

Makes ½ cup • Prep time: 15 minutes

Making your own mustard is quick, easy, and fun. Many of the recipes in this book call for mustard, so you could substitute your own homemade mustard for the commercial variety. This recipe gets an extra nutrition boost from the inclusion of turmeric. And you know it's low in sodium.

¼ cup dry mustard

3 tablespoons mustard seeds

3 tablespoons apple cider vinegar

3 tablespoons water

2 tablespoons freshly squeezed lemon juice

½ teaspoon turmeric

1. Combine the dry mustard, mustard seeds, vinegar, water, lemon juice, and turmeric in a jar with a tight-fitting lid and stir to combine.

2. Refrigerate the mustard for 3 days, stirring once a day and adding a bit more water every day if necessary.

3. After three days, the mustard is ready to use. You can process the mixture in a food processor or blender if you'd like smoother mustard. Refrigerate up to 2 weeks.

Ingredient Tip: The longer you store and stir the mustard before using it, the milder it will be. Mustard seed contains sulfur, a very aromatic, volatile compound that will be reduced as the mustard sits. Every time you stir the mustard, it releases more sulfur.

Nutrition Info per 1-Tablespoon Serving: Calories: 9; Total fat: 0g; Saturated fat: 0g; Sodium: 0mg; Potassium: 16mg; Phosphorus: 13mg; Carbohydrates: 1g; Fiber: 0g; Protein: 0g; Sugar: 0g

Cranberry Ketchup

DIABETES-FRIENDLY, LOW PROTEIN

Makes 1 cup • Prep time: 10 minutes • Cook time: 20 minutes

Did you know that ketchup used to be made with mushrooms, celery, and even fruit? Bottled ketchup tends to be high in sodium, sugar, and potassium. This recipe provides an alternative option using cranberries; there are no tomatoes in this ketchup. It's spicy and tangy with a slightly sweet flavor.

2 cups fresh cranberries

1⅓ cups water

3 tablespoons brown sugar

Juice of 1 lemon

2 teaspoons yellow mustard

¼ teaspoon onion powder

Pinch salt

Pinch ground cloves

1. Stir together the cranberries, water, brown sugar, lemon juice, mustard, onion powder, salt, and cloves in a medium saucepan over medium heat and bring to a boil.

2. Reduce the heat to low and simmer until the cranberries have popped, about 15 minutes.

3. Use an immersion blender or potato masher to mash the ingredients right in the saucepan.

4. After mashing, simmer the ketchup another 5 minutes until thickened.

5. Let the ketchup cool for 1 hour in the saucepan, then put into an airtight container and store in the refrigerator up to 1 week.

Ingredient Tip: Fresh cranberries are available in the fall and winter, so buy several bags and freeze them for later use in recipes.

Nutrition Info per 1-Tablespoon Serving: Calories: 13; Total fat: 0g; Saturated fat: 0g; Sodium: 19mg; Potassium: 17mg; Phosphorus: 3mg; Carbohydrates: 3g; Fiber: 1g; Protein: 0g; Sugar: 2g

Barbecue Sauce

DIABETES-FRIENDLY, LOW PROTEIN

Makes 2 cups • Prep time: 13 minutes • Cook time: 17 minutes

Store-bought barbecue sauce typically provides upward of 175 milligrams of sodium in just one serving. This recipe is flavorful without being too salty. If you're restricting potassium, you may be concerned about the inclusion of diced tomatoes in this recipe. Don't worry; the total potassium is low as long as you stick to the recommended serving size.

1 (14-ounce) can no-salt-added diced tomatoes, with juice

1 cup cherry tomatoes, cut in half

⅓ cup shredded carrots

3 tablespoons ketchup

2 tablespoons freshly squeezed lemon juice

1 tablespoon honey

2 teaspoons mustard

1 teaspoon paprika

½ teaspoon dried oregano

¼ teaspoon onion powder

⅛ teaspoon cayenne pepper

1. Combine the diced tomatoes, cherry tomatoes, carrots, ketchup, lemon juice, honey, mustard, paprika, oregano, onion powder, and cayenne in a medium saucepan over medium heat and bring to a boil.

2. Reduce the heat to low and simmer for 10 to 12 minutes or until the vegetables are tender.

3. Purée the mixture in a blender or food processor, or right in the saucepan using an immersion blender or a potato masher.

4. Return the mixture to the saucepan if using a blender or food processor. Bring to a simmer again.

5. Simmer the sauce for 5 minutes or until slightly thickened.

6. Cool the sauce for 1 hour in the saucepan, then store in the refrigerator in a container with a lid up to 2 weeks.

Ingredient Tip: Use freshly grated carrots in this recipe; don't buy pre-grated carrots because they are too hard to soften in 10 minutes.

Nutrition Info per 2-Tablespoon Serving: Calories: 15; Total fat: 0g; Saturated fat: 0g; Sodium: 38mg; Potassium: 94mg; Phosphorus: 10mg; Carbohydrates: 4g; Fiber: 1g; Protein: 0g; Sugar: 3g

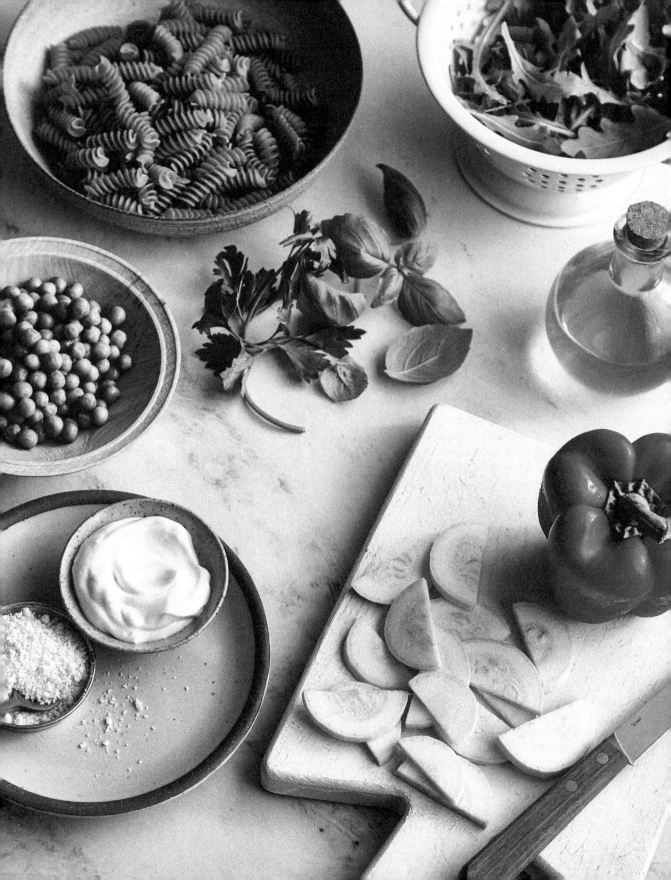

Food Lists for the Renal Diet

POTASSIUM

HIGHER POTASSIUM LEGUMES*

Greater than 300 mg per cooked ½-cup serving

Pinto beans

Lentils

Kidney beans

Black beans

LOWER POTASSIUM LEGUMES

Less than 300 mg per serving listed

¼ cup chopped peanuts

4 ounces tofu

½ cup chickpeas

2 tablespoons peanut butter

HIGHER POTASSIUM NUTS

Greater than 200 mg per ¼-cup serving

Pistachios (shelled)

Brazil nuts

Cashews

Pine nuts

Almonds

LOWER POTASSIUM NUTS

Less than 200mg per ¼-cup serving

Pecans

Walnuts

Macadamia nuts

HIGHER POTASSIUM SEAFOOD

Greater than 300 mg per cooked 3-ounce serving (unless otherwise specified)

Salmon

Trout

Sardines

Atlantic mackerel

Tilapia

4 clams

4 raw oysters

LOWER POTASSIUM SEAFOOD

Less than 300 mg per cooked 3-ounce serving (unless otherwise specified)

Cod

Sea bass

Scallops

Shrimp

Crab

Lobster

Sole

Flounder

* These higher potassium legumes can fit into a low-potassium diet as long as you stick to the serving size and avoid combining with higher-potassium vegetables, grains, and/or meat, poultry, or fish.

HIGHER POTASSIUM MEAT, POULTRY & EGGS

Greater than 300mg per cooked 3-ounce serving (unless otherwise specified)

Pork chop	Pork tenderloin	Steak

LOWER POTASSIUM MEAT, POULTRY & EGGS

Less than 300mg per cooked 3-ounce serving (unless otherwise specified)

Veal	Turkey breast	3 egg whites
Lamb	Chicken breast	2 eggs
Hamburger	Chicken thigh	

HIGHER POTASSIUM DAIRY & DAIRY ALTERNATIVE FOODS

Greater than 300mg per serving specified

1 cup evaporated milk	5-ounce container of	1 cup whole milk
1 cup low-fat milk	low-fat, plain yogurt	1 cup soy milk

LOWER POTASSIUM DAIRY & DAIRY ALTERNATIVE FOODS

Less than 300mg per serving specified

5-ounce container of low-fat, plain Greek yogurt	5-ounce container of whole-milk, Greek yogurt	½ cup chocolate ice cream
5-ounce container of whole-milk, plain yogurt	5 ounces almond-milk-based plain yogurt	1 cup almond milk
1 cup rice milk, unenriched	5 ounces cottage cheese	½ cup vanilla ice cream
		1 ounce cheese (most types)

HIGHER POTASSIUM GRAINS & STARCHES (MG)**

Greater than 200mg per cooked 1-cup serving (unless otherwise specified)

1 boiled skinless medium white potato**	1 boiled skinless medium sweet potato**	Quinoa

LOWER POTASSIUM GRAINS & STARCHES (MG)

Less than 200mg per cooked 1-cup serving (unless otherwise specified)

Steel cut oats	Wild rice	Polenta
2 medium slices whole-wheat bread	Pearled barley	2 medium slices rye bread
Bulgur	Old-fashioned oats	Couscous
Peas	1 whole-wheat English muffin	Spaghetti
Brown rice	Whole-wheat spaghetti	White rice

**High-potassium root vegetables, such as potatoes, can be double boiled to reduce their potassium content. Simply peel, slice, and dice your potatoes and place in boiling water for 15 minutes. Drain, add fresh water, and cook until done.

LOWER POTASSIUM FRUITS (MG)

Less than 200mg per ½ cup fresh, canned, or 1 small fruit (unless otherwise specified)

Apple

Applesauce

Apricot (fresh)

Berries

Cherries

Clementine

Dried apples, blueberries,
  cherries, or cranberries
  (¼ cup)

Fruit cup: any fruit,
  fruit cocktail

Grapes

Lemon or lime

Pear

Pineapple

Plums

Tangerine or
  mandarin orange

Watermelon (1 cup)

HIGHER POTASSIUM FRUITS (MG)

More than 200mg per ½ cup fresh, canned, or 1 small fruit (unless otherwise specified)

Avocado

Banana

Dried fruit: raisins, dates,
  figs, apricots, bananas,
  peaches, pears, or
  prunes (¼ cup)

Honeydew

Kiwi

Nectarine

Orange

Papaya

Peach

Plantain

Pomegranate

LOWER POTASSIUM VEGETABLES (MG)

Less than 200mg per 1 cup leafy greens or ½ cup fresh, cooked, or canned vegetables (unless otherwise specified)

Alfalfa sprouts

Asparagus

Bamboo shoots (canned)

Bean sprouts

Beets (canned)

Broccoli

Cabbage

Carrots

Cauliflower

Celery

Cucumber

Eggplant

Green or wax beans

Greens: collard, mustard,
  or turnip

Jicama/yam bean

Kale

Lettuce: all types

Mushrooms
  (raw or canned)

Okra

Onion or leek

Peas: green, sugar snap,
  or snow

Peppers: green, red,
  or yellow

Radish

Rhubarb

Spinach (raw)

Spaghetti squash

Cherry tomatoes

Turnip

Yellow summer squash

Water chestnuts (canned)

More than 200mg per 1 cup leafy greens or ½ cup fresh, cooked, or canned vegetables (unless otherwise specified)

Acorn squash

Artichoke

Beet greens

Brussels sprouts

Butternut squash

Chard (cooked)

Chinese cabbage (cooked)

Corn (1 ear)

Edamame

Hubbard squash

Kohlrabi

Lentils

Parsnips

Potatoes

Pumpkins

Rutabaga

Spinach (cooked)

Tomatoes

Tomato sauce, tomato
  paste, tomato juice

Yams

Zucchini

Vegetable juice

PROTEIN

Protein-rich foods include meat, poultry, fish, eggs, milk, cheese, legumes, nuts, and grains. Fruits and vegetables contain very low amounts of protein and are therefore not included.

Per ½-cup serving cooked (unless otherwise specified)

Soybeans 16

4 ounces silken tofu 10,
  not silken 15

Lentils 9

¼ cup peanuts 9

Pinto beans 8

Kidney beans 8

Black beans 8

Chickpeas 7

2 tablespoons peanut
  butter 7

Per ¼-cup serving (unless otherwise specified)

Almonds 7

Cashews 6

Pistachios 6

Walnuts 5

Brazil nuts 5

Pine nuts 4

Pecans 3

Macadamia nuts 2

PROTEIN IN GRAINS & STARCHES (G)

Per 1-cup serving cooked (unless otherwise specified)

2 medium slices
   whole-wheat bread 9

Quinoa 8

Peas 8

Whole-wheat or regular
   spaghetti 8

Steel-cut oats 7

Wild rice 7

Old-fashioned oats 6

Brown rice 6

Bulgur 6

Couscous 6

Whole-wheat English
   muffin 6

2 medium slices
   rye bread 5

Pearled barley 5

Polenta/grits 4

White Rice 4

PROTEIN IN SEAFOOD (G)

Per 3-ounce serving cooked (unless otherwise specified)

Sardines 22

Salmon 22

Tilapia 22

Shrimp 20

Atlantic mackerel 20

Trout 20

Sea bass 20

Scallops 18

Cod 17

4 raw oysters 17

Lobster 16

Crab 15

Sole 13

Flounder 13

4 clams 12

PROTEIN IN MEAT, POULTRY & EGGS (G)

Per 3-ounce serving cooked (unless otherwise specified)

Turkey breast 26

Chicken breast 26

Pork chop 25

Steak 25

Chicken thigh 24

Pork tenderloin 24

Lamb 24

Hamburger 22

Veal 21

2 eggs 13

3 egg whites 11

PROTEIN IN DAIRY & DAIRY ALTERNATIVE FOODS (G)

Per 1-cup serving (unless otherwise specified)

1 cup evaporated milk 17

5 ounces low-fat cottage
   cheese 15

5-ounce container of
   low-fat, plain Greek
   yogurt 15

5-ounce container of
   whole-milk, Greek
   yogurt 13

1 ounce cheese (most
   types) 6-8

1 cup low-fat milk 8

1 cup whole milk 8

1 cup soy milk 8

5-ounce container of
   low-fat, plain yogurt 7

5 ounces almond-milk-
   based plain yogurt 6

5-ounce container of
   whole-milk, plain
   yogurt 5

½ cup ice cream 3

1 cup rice milk,
   unenriched 2

1 cup rice milk,
   unenriched 2

1 cup almond milk 1

SODIUM

Check food labels for actual sodium content per serving

Table salt

Most canned foods (unless specified as no-salt-added or low-sodium)

Bread

Seasoning salt

Ham

Sauerkraut

Soy sauce

Sausage

Fast foods

Teriyaki sauce

Microwave meals

Salad dressings

Garlic salt

Potato chips

Hot dogs

Onion salt

Salted crackers

Cold cuts, deli meat

Spam

Buttermilk

Corned beef

Vegetable juices

Canned ravioli

Frozen prepared foods

Barbecue sauce

Bouillon cubes

Bacon

Smoked fish

Baking mixes (pancakes, desserts)

Steak sauce

Monosodium glutamate (MSG)

Ketchup

High-sodium cereals

Check food labels for actual sodium content per serving

Fresh garlic

Low-sodium salad dressings

Canned food with no added salt

Fresh onion

Allspice

Low-sodium seasoning blends

Black pepper

Ginger

Fresh fish

Lemon juice

Rosemary

Eggs

Vinegar, regular or flavored

Thyme

Dry mustard

Nuts, unsalted

Unsalted popcorn

Sage

Pretzels, unsalted

Homemade or no-salt-added broth

Tarragon

Crackers, unsalted

Lower-sodium breads and cereals (check label)

Dill

PHOSPHORUS

Phosphorus is found in protein-rich foods. Fruits and vegetables contain very low amounts of phosphorus and are therefore not included. Tables include total phosphorus and phosphorus adjusted for estimated bioavailability in descending order.

Plant Sources of Phosphorus: Low Bioavailability
*Adjusted phosphorus was calculated using an estimate of 50-percent bioavailability of phosphorus in plant sources.

PHOSPHORUS IN LEGUMES (MG)
Per ½-cup serving cooked (unless otherwise specified)

FOOD	PHOSPHORUS	ADJUSTED PHOSPHORUS*
Soybeans	211	106
Lentils	178	89
Chickpeas	138	69
¼ cup peanuts	137	69
Pinto beans	126	63
Kidney beans	122	61
4 ounces tofu, not silken	122	61
Black beans	120	60
2 tablespoons peanut butter	108	54
4 ounces silken tofu	102	51

PHOSPHORUS IN NUTS (MG)
Per ¼-cup serving

FOOD	PHOSPHORUS	ADJUSTED PHOSPHORUS*
Brazil nuts	241	121
Pine nuts	194	97
Cashews	191	96
Almonds	156	78
Pistachios	151	76
Walnuts	101	51
Pecans	76	38
Macadamia nuts	63	32

FOOD	PHOSPHORUS	ADJUSTED PHOSPHORUS*
1 cup cooked quinoa	281	141
1 cup cooked steel-cut oats	219	110
1 cup cooked brown rice	208	104
1 cup cooked whole-wheat spaghetti	178	89
1 cup cooked old-fashioned oats	172	86
1 cup cooked wild rice	135	68
1 cup cooked bulgur	134	67
1 cup cooked pearled barley	121	61
1 cup cooked couscous	80	40
1 cup cooked polenta/grits	53	27

ANIMAL SOURCES OF PHOSPHORUS: MEDIUM BIOAVAILABILITY

*Adjusted phosphorus was calculated using an estimate of 70-percent bioavailability of phosphorus in animal sources.

PHOSPHORUS IN SEAFOOD (MG)

Per 3-ounce serving cooked (unless otherwise specified)

FOOD	PHOSPHORUS	ADJUSTED PHOSPHORUS*
Scallops	362	253
4 raw oysters	294	206
Sardines	272	190
Sole	263	184
Flounder	262	183
Atlantic mackerel	236	165
Trout	230	161
Salmon	218	153
Sea bass	211	148
Shrimp	202	141
Crab	199	139
Tilapia	174	122
4 clams	164	115
Lobster	157	81
Light tuna	139	97
Cod	117	82

Phosphorus Cooking Tip: Research shows that preparing meats by boiling them in liquid can reduce the phosphorus content by 10 to 50 percent. This works best when the meat is sliced before cooking. Because the phosphorus is leached into the liquid, you'll need to discard the cooking liquid before serving.

PHOSPHORUS IN MEAT, POULTRY & EGGS (G)

Per 3-ounce serving cooked (unless otherwise specified)

FOOD	PHOSPHORUS	ADJUSTED PHOSPHORUS*
Pork tenderloin	248	174
Steak	230	161
Turkey breast	196	137
Veal	190	133
Pork chop	189	132
Chicken breast	184	129
Chicken thigh	180	126
Lamb	173	121
Hamburger	158	111
2 eggs	172	120
3 egg whites	15	11

PHOSPHORUS IN DAIRY FOODS (G)

Per serving size listed

FOOD	PHOSPHORUS	ADJUSTED PHOSPHORUS*
1 cup evaporated milk	460	322
1 cup low-fat milk	225	158
5 ounces low-fat cottage cheese	213	149
1 cup whole milk	205	144
5-ounce container of low-fat, plain yogurt	204	143
5-ounce container of whole-milk, Greek yogurt	191	134
5-ounce container of low-fat, plain Greek yogurt	141	99
5-ounce container of whole-milk, plain yogurt	135	95
1 ounce cheese (most types)	130-180	91-126
1 ounce feta	96	67
1 ounce goat cheese	73	51
½ cup ice cream	69	48
1 ounce Brie	53	37

PROCESSED SOURCES OF PHOSPHORUS: HIGH BIOAVAILABILITY (80–100 PERCENT)

The food industry is not required to provide the phosphorus content of processed foods. Foods with phosphorus additives represent the most bioavailable form of phosphorus in the diet. The following foods frequently contain phosphorus additives. Always check the ingredients of foods to be sure.

Fast food ("fast-fresh" food may be okay)

Bottled drinks (such as soda, flavored waters, juices)

Certain brands of non-dairy creamers or half and half

Certain brands of non-dairy milks

Processed meats (includes all cold cuts, as well as breakfast meats such as sausage, bacon, and turkey bacon)

Frozen prepared meals

Many canned foods

Processed sweet and savory snack foods (cakes, cookies, cheese-based snacks)

HIGH-FIBER CARBOHYDRATES

Fiber is found in vegetables, fruits, whole grains, nuts, and legumes.

HIGH-FIBER LEGUMES (G)

Per ½-cup serving cooked (unless otherwise specified)

Pinto beans 8

Black beans 8

Kidney beans 6

Lentils 6

Chickpeas 5

HIGH-FIBER NUTS (G)

Per ¼-cup serving

Almonds 4

Brazil nuts 3

Pecans 3

Macadamia nuts 3

Pistachios 3

Per 1 cup cooked (unless otherwise specified)

Old-fashioned oats 8

Peas 7

Whole-wheat spaghetti 6

Bulgur 6

Steel-cut oats 5

Quinoa 5

1 medium sweet potato 4

1 medium white potato 4

2 medium slices
  whole-wheat bread 4

Whole-wheat English
  muffin 4

Brown rice 3

2 medium slices
  rye bread 3

per ½ cup fresh, canned, or 1 small fruit (unless otherwise specified)

Pear 6

Apple 4

Blackberries 4

Raspberries 4

Blueberries 2

Strawberries 2

¼ avocado 2

Mandarin orange 2

Per ½ cup cooked (unless otherwise specified)

Collard greens 4

Brussels sprouts 3

Broccoli 3

Asparagus 2

Carrots 2

Green beans 2

Mushrooms 2

1 cup raw baby spinach 1

Cauliflower 1

HEART-HEALTHY FATS

Olive oil

Avocado oil

Sesame oil

Flaxseed oil (keep
  refrigerated and do
  not heat)

Hemp oil (keep
  refrigerated and avoid
  high heat)

Sesame oil (keep
  refrigerated and avoid
  high heat)

Walnut oil (keep
  refrigerated and avoid
  high heat)

Atlantic mackerel (avoid
  king mackerel due to
  mercury content)

Salmon

Rainbow trout

Sardines

NUTS/NUT BUTTERS & SEEDS

Peanuts and peanut butter

Almonds and
almond butter

Walnuts

Cashews

Brazil nuts

Pine nuts

Pecans

Macadamia nuts

Pistachios

Sunflower seeds

Flax seeds

Chia Seeds

MISCELLANEOUS

Avocado

Low-sodium olives

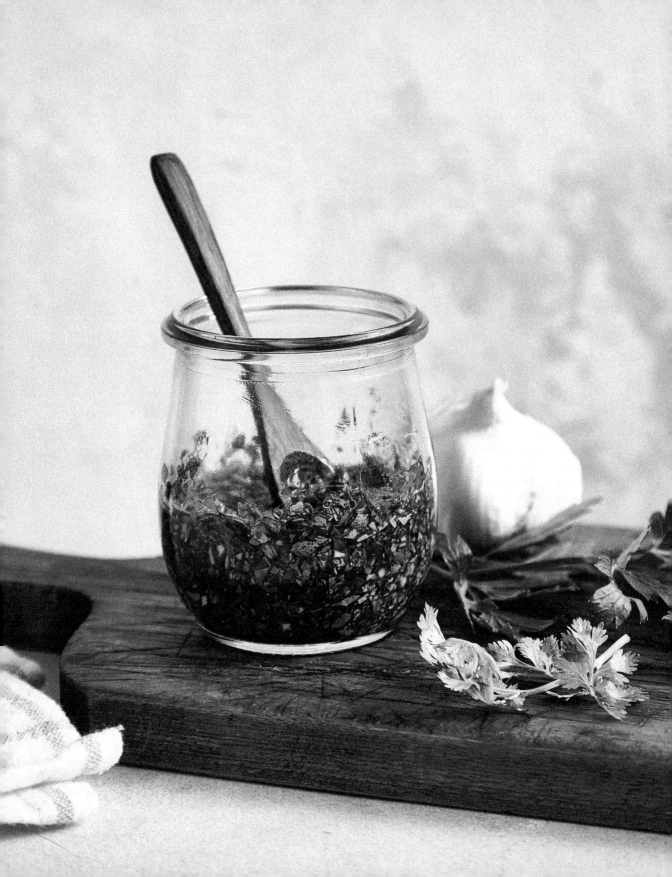

The Dirty Dozen™ and The Clean Fifteen™

A nonprofit environmental watchdog organization called Environmental Working Group (EWG) looks at data supplied by the US Department of Agriculture (USDA) and the Food and Drug Administration (FDA) about pesticide residues. Each year it compiles a list of the best and worst pesticide loads found in commercial crops. You can use these lists to decide which fruits and vegetables to buy organic to minimize your exposure to pesticides and which produce is considered safe enough to buy conventionally. This does not mean they are pesticide-free, though, so wash these fruits and vegetables thoroughly. The list is updated annually, and you can find it online at EWG.org/FoodNews.

DIRTY DOZEN™

1. strawberries
2. spinach
3. kale
4. nectarines
5. apples
6. grapes
7. peaches
8. cherries
9. pears
10. tomatoes
11. celery
12. potatoes

CLEAN FIFTEEN™

1. avocados
2. sweet corn*
3. pineapples
4. sweet peas (frozen)
5. onions
6. papayas*
7. eggplants
8. asparagus
9. kiwis
10. cabbages
11. cauliflower
12. cantaloupes
13. broccoli
14. mushrooms
15. honeydew melons

* A small amount of sweet corn, papaya, and summer squash sold in the United States is produced from genetically modified seeds. Buy organic varieties of these crops if you want to avoid genetically modified produce.

Measurement Conversions

	US STANDARD	US STANDARD (OUNCES)	METRIC (APPROXIMATE)
VOLUME EQUIVALENTS (LIQUID)	2 tablespoons	1 fl. oz.	30 mL
	¼ cup	2 fl. oz.	60 mL
	½ cup	4 fl. oz.	120 mL
	1 cup	8 fl. oz.	240 mL
	1½ cups	12 fl. oz.	355 mL
	2 cups or 1 pint	16 fl. oz.	475 mL
	4 cups or 1 quart	32 fl. oz.	1 L
	1 gallon	128 fl. oz.	4 L
VOLUME EQUIVALENTS (DRY)	⅛ teaspoon		0.5 mL
	¼ teaspoon		1 mL
	½ teaspoon		2 mL
	¾ teaspoon		4 mL
	1 teaspoon		5 mL
	1 tablespoon		15 mL
	¼ cup		59 mL
	⅓ cup		79 mL
	½ cup		118 mL
	⅔ cup		156 mL
	¾ cup		177 mL
	1 cup		235 mL
	2 cups or 1 pint		475 mL
	3 cups		700 mL
	4 cups or 1 quart		1 L
	½ gallon		2 L
	1 gallon		4 L
WEIGHT EQUIVALENTS	½ ounce		15 g
	1 ounce		30 g
	2 ounces		60 g
	4 ounces		115 g
	8 ounces		225 g
	12 ounces		340 g
	16 ounces or 1 pound		455 g

	FAHRENHEIT (F)	CELSIUS (C) (APPROXIMATE)
OVEN TEMPERATURES	250°F	120°F
	300°F	150°C
	325°F	180°C
	375°F	190°C
	400°F	200°C
	425°F	220°C
	450°F	230°C

Index

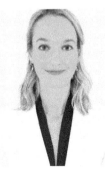

Aisling Whelan, MS, RDN, CDN is a registered dietitian who uses a whole-person, whole-food-based approach to help clients reclaim their health and improve their quality of life. She completed her didactic program in dietetics at Simmons University in Boston and obtained a master's degree in clinical nutrition from New York University. Aisling has extensive experience working with the chronic kidney disease population. Her first introduction to renal nutrition began when she worked as a dietitian in a hemodialysis facility. In this role, Aisling was surprised to learn that most of her patients had never met with a dietitian prior to starting dialysis. It was this discovery that inspired Aisling to start her own private practice specializing in nutrition therapy for pre-dialysis CKD patients. Aisling is passionate about empowering her patients to implement realistic and sustainable changes aimed at slowing down the progression of their kidney disease. She also continues to work with dialysis patients who wish to improve their health and reduce the risk of further complications. In addition to specializing in kidney disease, Aisling also has expertise in treating other conditions such as diabetes, obesity, hypertension, and women's health issues. Aisling lives with her husband in New York City.

CPSIA information can be obtained
at www.ICGtesting.com
Printed in the USA
LVHW070000081120
670941LV00002B/2

9 781641 526968